Everyday Guide to Managing Your Medicines

Jack E. Fincham, PhD, RPh
Professor
Department of Pharmacy Practice
School of Pharmacy
Health Sciences Building
University of Missouri-Kansas City
Kansas City, Missouri

JONES AND BARTLETT PUBLISHERS
Sudbury, Massachusetts
BOSTON   TORONTO   LONDON   SINGAPORE

World Headquarters
Jones and Bartlett Publishers
40 Tall Pine Drive
Sudbury, MA 01776
978-443-5000
info@jbpub.com
www.jbpub.com

Jones and Bartlett Publishers
Canada
6339 Ormindale Way
Mississauga, Ontario L5V 1J2
Canada

Jones and Bartlett Publishers
International
Barb House, Barb Mews
London W6 7PA
United Kingdom

Jones and Bartlett's books and products are available through most bookstores and online booksellers. To contact Jones and Bartlett Publishers directly, call 800-832-0034, fax 978-443-8000, or visit our website www.jbpub.com.

Substantial discounts on bulk quantities of Jones and Bartlett's publications are available to corporations, professional associations, and other qualified organizations. For details and specific discount information, contact the special sales department at Jones and Bartlett via the above contact information or send an email to specialsales@jbpub.com.

The authors, editor, and publisher have made every effort to provide accurate information. However, they are not responsible for errors, omissions, or for any outcomes related to the use of the contents of this book and take no responsibility for the use of the products and procedures described. Treatments and side effects described in this book may not be applicable to all people; likewise, some people may require a dose or experience a side effect that is not described herein. Drugs and medical devices are discussed that may have limited availability controlled by the Food and Drug Administration (FDA) for use only in a research study or clinical trial. Research, clinical practice, and government regulations often change the accepted standard in this field. When consideration is being given to use of any drug in the clinical setting, the health care provider or reader is responsible for determining FDA status of the drug, reading the package insert, and reviewing prescribing information for the most up-to-date recommendations on dose, precautions, and contraindications, and determining the appropriate usage for the product. This is especially important in the case of drugs that are new or seldom used.

Library of Congress Cataloging-in-Publication Data
Fincham, Jack E.
  Everyday guide to managing your medicines / Jack Fincham.
    p. cm.
  ISBN-13: 978-0-7637-5101-2
  ISBN-10: 0-7637-5101-4
  1. Drugs—Popular works. 2. Pharmacology—Popular works. I. Title.
  RM301.15.F56 2008
  615'.1—dc22
                                    2007013275
6048

Production Credits
Executive Editor: David Cella
Editorial Assistant: Lisa Gordon
Production Director: Amy Rose
Production Editor: Renée Sekerak
Associate Marketing Manager: Jennifer Bengtson
Manufacturing and Inventory Coordinator: Amy Bacus
Cover Design: Kristin E. Ohlin
Composition: Auburn Associates, Inc.
Printing and Binding: Malloy Incorporated
Cover Printing: Malloy Incorporated

Printed in the United States of America
11 10 09 08 07   10 9 8 7 6 5 4 3 2 1

To Meadow and all who helped to bring her to us, and to all those associated with Springer Spaniel Rescue Programs.

CONTENTS

Chapter 11 Complementary and Alternative Medicine 115

Chapter 12 Antibiotics 125

CHAPTER ONE

Introduction

Each of us can use help with our drug-taking needs. We can also use more information about our health conditions or disease states. Even doctors, nurses, and pharmacists struggle to take prescriptions as they should. Often, health professionals ask that you "do as I say and not as I do." It is human nature to struggle with medicine-taking requirements. It is also hard to be unbiased about diseases that you might have. It is normal to feel differently about your health and health status because it is very personal and very private. This book will help you understand basic medication-taking needs and will provide you with information about some common diseases that you or your loved ones might have. Also, there is a chapter on complementary and alternative medicine that you will find informative.

Doctors spend years and years studying drugs; pharmacists spend 6 years studying drugs before becoming eligible for state licensure. However, you are expected to know about drugs *without* a lot of information provided to you. The fruits of all the study by your health providers are not beneficial if you, the most important person in health care, do not know about your drugs, their use, and other associated information.

Nothing presented in this book is meant to take the place of anything that your caregivers provide to you or suggest you do. This book is meant to be a complement and supplement to other health information that you receive from any number of sources. You should always check with your doctor about information that you receive that may affect your health or is related to your disease conditions.

There are two appendices at the end of this book:

- Appendix A—Websites for Senior Citizen Information
- Appendix B—Websites for More Information About Drugs

These compilations are in the book to provide you with resources and several places that you can go to find more information about drugs. Appendix A provides internet sites that can help seniors with different needs and requirements. Appendix B lists numerous Internet sites that can help you understand more about drugs and herbs.

Some of the information covered in this book may affect you more than others. However, some of it is important for everyone to know, such as the information about prescription and over-the-counter (OTC) drugs. Often, it is assumed that people know things about drugs or their classification, but this is not always the case. This is the reason this book has been written. It is meant to help answer your everyday drug-taking questions. It is also meant to provide you with help that you might not always be able to find elsewhere.

General topics covered in this book include:

- Understanding drugs and their use
- What your caregivers need to know about your health
- Dos and don'ts of drugs
- Tips to enhance compliance with your medications
- Getting your drugs and drug taking in order
- Over-the-counter pain relief drugs
- Drug–drug interactions
- Drug–herbal product interactions
- Complementary and alternative medicine
- Antibiotics
- Resources available to help you with Medicare Part D
- Other resources to help you with Medicare
- Issues that currently affect everyday medicine taking

Above all else, my hope in writing this book is to have you become the very best patient that you can be. This includes knowing as much as you can about drugs, the type of drugs available, and how to take them in the best fashion possible. This knowledge also includes understanding how to deal with side effects and what to do if your drugs do not work.

Read along, learn what you can, and realize you can always achieve a better state of health and well-being!

CHAPTER TWO

What Your Caregivers Need to Know about Your Health

Introduction

You cannot always assume that those that provide care for you know everything they should about your health. If you see multiple doctors, and most of us do, they do not always share as much information as they should. The same holds true with different pharmacies that you might use for prescriptions. Pharmacies do not routinely share information about your records unless you ask them to. Always err on the side of caution, and let those who treat you know as much about your health as possible. This chapter will provide you with some tips on how to keep your own medical records. What you need to tell those who care for you will also be discussed. Always tell your doctors as much as you can about your health and health history. The more your caregivers know about your health, the better position they are in to provide the best care for you.

It Is Important to Provide Information to Your Care Providers

Your health information needs to be shared with all those who provide care for you. So, your nurses, pharmacists, and others who provide healthcare services to you need to know as much about your health as possible.

Most of the information on your doctor's medical record is from the care that you have received while a patient with that doctor. These records may not be thorough enough to cover your past medical care. Other doctors' care that you have received in the past may not be recorded in your current doctor's record of care provided to you. You may also be seeing several doctors at the same time:

- Your regular doctor
- A specialist or two
- Other care providers

Because not all of your former medical care treatments may be listed in each of the doctor's individual records, you must let them know of your previous treatments.

In Some Cases, Your Doctor Will Have Records from Your Past Healthcare Providers

Usually, this does not happen unless you yourself have asked for records from all your previous providers. Then perhaps you have given the doctor what you have collected. There may be a charge for you to obtain your records from previous doctors. But you also should know that, even if you cannot afford to pay the fee to obtain your records, the records still must be provided to you.

You may be the best person to maintain your medical records from many sources. If so, you may also have someone in your family help you with this. These records belong to you, and you should safeguard them like you would any of your valuable possessions.

MULTIPLE DOCTORS

If you are seen by multiple doctors, your medical records may or may not be complete enough to include your medical history from all doctors that you see. Not all doctors talk to each other as they should. Your doctor may refer you to a specialist for care but may not always receive the records from the other physician. They certainly should, but sometimes, this may not happen. Or, records may not be placed in your file.

HOSPITAL RECORDS

Sometimes your records from a hospital stay are not always shared with all of your doctors. The referring doctor or the doctor who admits you will receive a letter about your stay. However, it would be rare for the complete record to be provided unless you are the one who provides the record to your doctor. It would also be unusual for one hospital to provide information from your stay to another hospital. You or your doctor would have to provide this information to the other hospital.

The organization that oversees the quality of healthcare services provided from hospitals, the Joint Commission on Accreditation of Health Care Organizations (www.jointcommission.org), understands that this lack of sharing of medical information is a problem. When we are dismissed from a hospital, the last thing we normally think about is making sure we take our medical records with us. You can contact the hospital later to obtain this information. I would encourage you to do this.

KEEPING YOUR OWN RECORDS

If you have a computer, you can also store medical information and keep the material updated. This type of a record is not as complete as your doctor's medical records, but it will allow you to track the major segments of your care. It will also allow you to provide this information to your caregivers. It should be secured on your computer. If you do not have a computer or do not feel like you can accomplish this, do not worry. You might have a family member who would be more than happy to assist you.

See Figure 2-1 for a spreadsheet example of a medical record that you can store on your computer. This particular record in Figure 2-1 is from the Microsoft Excel spreadsheet program. If you do not have a computer or access to one, you can write this information down by hand and keep it in a place where you will always know where it is. You can add and delete information as necessary either by hand or on the computer.

Immunization History

In Figure 2-1, there is a subheading titled "Immunization History" and a section for listing the immunizations that you have received. This would be the place where you would record your immunizations, such as:

- Flu shots
- Pneumonia vaccine (pneumococcal pneumonia)
- Hepatitis vaccines
- Tetanus

My Health Record

Name ....

Birth Date ....

Medical Plan ....

Medical Plan ID ....

Emergency Contact Name ....

Address ....

Phone ....

Alternate Phone ....

Immunization History

Date	Type

Known Medical Conditions/Allergies

Name	Description

Medications

Name	Description	Dosage

Medical Visits

Date	Description	Attending Physician	Diagnosis	Tests Performed	Test Results	Prescribed Action	Prescribed Medication	Notes

Figure 2-1   Medical record form.

9

- Diphtheria
- Pertussis
- Others

By using this system (or perhaps another system), you will be able to remember when and where you received these shots and to provide your caregivers with this information. It will be very useful for you to keep track of this information for yourself as well as for others providing care for you.

Medical Conditions and Allergies

Also depicted in Figure 2-1 is a section where you list your known medical conditions and allergies. It is important that you list your medical conditions. It is also crucial to list what allergies you have. Please do not assume that because you once told someone your allergy history, that they will remember it. Always provide this information. Keeping track of this information on a sheet such as the one depicted in Figure 2-1 or on a computer will be helpful to you and to others providing care for you. It is also important that someone in your family also know this information. If, in the unfortunate event that you are admitted to a hospital and not able to speak for yourself, it will be invaluable if someone has this information and can provide it to workers in the hospital.

Adverse Drug Reactions

When you see your doctors for regular appointments, always let them know about any adverse drug reactions that you have had in the past. Often when you are seen in the office, a nurse will see you first. They may take your blood pressure, ask you to be weighed, and take your temperature. During this time with the nurse, always let him or her know about your drug allergies. When you are asked by your doctor about what drugs you might be allergic to, always provide this information. Do not hesitate to tell the doctor this information at every visit.

When you are hospitalized, always tell everyone who takes care of you about your history of allergies to medications or previous adverse drug reactions. Have your family members or friends let the caregivers know this information as well. You will have a chart on the floor where your hospital room is located; make sure this allergy information is included in this record. Please do not assume that everyone will know this information just because you may have told one of the people who care for you.

Your Previous Medical Visits

A portion of the form in Figure 2-1 provides a space for you to write information about your medical visits to doctors. The headings in this form will help you remember what you have been seen for, and it will be helpful if you take this information with you when you are seen by another doctor. It is important for you to record when you see a doctor and what you were seen for. The visit might be for a routine follow-up, a sinus infection, a sore on your hand, etc. The information does not need to be written in medical jargon; you can use your own words to document the facts of the visit, such as:

- Who was the doctor?
- What was the diagnosis?
- Were there any tests performed?
- What was the result of the test or tests?
- What was the action the doctor suggested?
- What drugs were prescribed?

Indicate what you thought of the visit in the section titled "Notes." These are your notes and thoughts about the visit and what happened during and afterward. You should note all of the doctors that you have seen. This includes those who you see now and those who you have seen in the past. Note the specialists, such as eye doctors and others, who provide care to you. After you note this in your records, you will be in a better position to let your caregivers know as much information as possible about your current and past care. Recording information such as this will allow you to remember aspects of your care. It will also make it easier to indicate to others what you have been treated for in the past. Keep this information as current as you can, and continue to add to the list. If you are starting this record from scratch, it may take some time to write all of the information down. However, this record will help both you and your doctors move forward. Again, the more information that is available to your caregivers, the better position they are in to provide you with the best care possible.

Your Current Medications and Supplements

Also provided in Figure 2-1 is a place to write down the medications that you currently take. It is very important for you to complete this drug history as thoroughly as possible. Again, the drug history is a list of the drugs and medicines that you are currently taking; this information is important to provide to your caregivers. It helps them to continue to prescribe or dispense a drug that you already take and allows them to establish what drugs you do not take that might be helpful to you. This listing will give your doctors and pharmacists an idea of your medications and intended effects. You may be taking substances, such as supplements or herbs, that you do not view as drugs. These substances can have health effects and may inhibit other drugs. Conversely, they may also make a drug work too well and lead to an adverse effect.

Your caregivers need to know what you are taking for your health. Let's consider what you should put on this list. You should list the drugs that you take for chronic health problems. Examples of medications for chronic conditions include high blood pressure medications, drug or insulin injections for diabetes, and drugs for heart failure. You might also be taking an antibiotic or a drug to treat your allergies. In addition, keep a list of drugs that you have taken in the past. If listing all of these current and former drugs seems overwhelming, ask your pharmacist to help you by printing out from the pharmacy computer a listing of drugs you have taken in the past and drugs you are taking now. If you use more than one pharmacy, obtain this information from all of your pharmacies. List every medication that you take that has been prescribed for you by your doctors.

This list should also include drugs that you take occasionally but not every day. Here you should list all of the drugs that you take for which you do not need a prescription. Be as thorough as you can. Include these drugs in the drug history because, even though you may not need a prescription for them, they are drugs just the same. You may be buying these drugs from a grocery store, a super center, and/or from a community chain or independent pharmacy. You should list the various supplements that you take. You may take a multivitamin (containing many vitamins) or a multivitamin that contains minerals. These minerals can include iron, calcium, zinc, etc.

Social Drugs That You Might Take

There are other substances that normally would not be called a drug, but these need to be included in a drug history as well, including:

- Coffee
- Tea
- Cigarettes or tobacco in any form (for many reasons, please stop smoking if you smoke!)

Each of these substances can influence the medication that you take. There is a very long list of drugs that are adversely affected by smoking. They include:

- Pain relief medications
- Drugs for high blood pressure
- Drugs to treat diabetes
- Drugs like warfarin, a drug used to thin your blood
- Numerous other drugs

You also need to inform your doctor and caregivers if you consume alcoholic beverages (e.g., beer, wine, liquor). You need to indicate how many drinks you consume over a period of time (days, weeks, or months). Alcohol may also impact numerous drugs that you may be taking.

Information That You Can Obtain
from Your Pharmacy or Pharmacies

If you have numerous pharmacies that you use for your prescription medications, you will need to have each of them supply you with a listing of the drug you take. Each pharmacy has a sophisticated computer system, but this information is not shared between pharmacies. Therefore, the prescriptions that you obtain from each pharmacy will need to be consolidated. You can take the information from each pharmacy that you frequent and merge the information into one list. Obviously if you obtain all of your medications from one pharmacy, only that pharmacy will have a history of your prescriptions. The pharmacies will not have records of the over-the-counter drugs that you take, so you will need to add this information to your list. The complete list of the drugs that you take will be very helpful for those providing care to you.

Also note the herbal remedies that you might take for various reasons. Some of these herbal products will adversely affect the prescription drugs that you take. It may make them work less effectively or may actually cause adverse effects. It is always best to ask your pharmacist and your doctor to help guide you on which of these products you can take safely with the other drugs that you are taking.

Help Your Doctors to Help You!

Let your doctors know about all of your allergies. Allergies can be to a medicine, a certain food, or plants. Make a note of these allergies in a place where you will always remember where the information is, and let those who provide care to you understand what the severity of the allergies might be.

I have listed items that you need to let your doctor know about. However, there are a series of important questions that you need to ask your doctor about the drugs he or she prescribes. These questions include:

- What am I being treated for?
- What does this drug do?
- Will it interfere with other drugs?
- When will it start to work?
- Are there any side effects?

- Will it work?
- Do I take it with food?
- Do I take it on an empty stomach?
- Should I take it before or after meals?
- How long will I need to take this drug?
- Does it take the place of other drugs that I am taking?

Feel free to let your doctor know what you expect from treatments. Often we may feel reluctant to ask doctors questions such as these. However, you need to ask these questions; it is your right, and you should be able to have input in your medical care plans. Do you have a preference for taking a certain drug? If so, let your doctor know. Also let the doctor know the bad reactions you may have experienced with certain drugs in the past.

HAVE OTHERS HELP YOU

Sometimes you will need to have others help you with providing information to caregivers. This situation may occur when you are seen in an emergency situation and simply cannot tell others about your health condition. You may be hospitalized and unable to talk with those providing care for you in the institution. You also may be too sick to let others know about your health and medical care history. In these cases, ask a family member or friend to help you by providing this information to others for you.

Summary

To summarize, let all of your caregivers know as much as possible about your health. Each provider needs to know all of the drugs you take. Also let each of your caregivers know about the drugs you have taken in the past that have caused you to have bad reactions and about your drug allergies.

CHAPTER THREE

General Information about Drugs

Introduction

Throughout this book, the terms drug and medication will be used interchangeably. When I use the word drug in this context, it is in reference to a legitimate medication used for therapeutic purposes. The purpose of this chapter is to acquaint you with some general information about drugs and their use. If you have any questions about your drugs and their use, always feel free to ask your pharmacist, doctor, or nurse. Even if you do not have your prescriptions filled at a particular pharmacy, you can always ask a pharmacist a question about drugs.

Drugs Are Modern Miracles

It was not until the mid-20th century that drugs manufactured on a large scale became commonplace and drugs were widely used. The advent of the new age of pharmacy was ushered in shortly after World War II when the antibiotic penicillin was mass produced and introduced for widespread use. Later, the introduction of drugs such as chlorpromazine in the early 1960s, which was used to treat mental disorders (e.g., psychoses, psychotic episodes), revolutionized the treatment of the mentally ill in the United States and throughout the world. Also in the 1960s, the entry of the drug levodopa into the marketplace revolutionized the treatment of Parkinson's disease. Drugs to treat heart ailments, cancer, diabetes, and infectious disease are much in demand. As the demand for pharmaceuticals has risen, so have the prices and profits of the pharmaceutical industry. It is not uncommon for the percent increase in the price of drugs to rise by double digits each year. Drugs are available to treat many chronic conditions. There are many older and newer drugs that are available to treat conditions.

Classes of Drugs in the United States

Currently, in the United States, there are two classes of medications, prescription and nonprescription, or so-called over-the-counter (OTC), drugs. Any new drug can be submitted for approval as a prescription or OTC medication. However, virtually all new drugs in the United States enter the market as a prescription drug product. After use of the drug occurs over a period of years, the manufacturing company can petition the U.S. Food and Drug Administration (FDA) to switch the product from prescription to OTC status. This happens on a regular basis.

Again, the two basic types of drugs are:

- Prescription drugs, which require a prescription to be written by your doctor
- Over-the-counter drugs, which can be purchased without a prescription at many different places

Drugs in both of these categories are medicines and should be taken with care. Just because a drug can be bought without a prescription does not mean that it is not a real medicine. Nonprescription drugs should be used cautiously, just like prescription medicines.

U.S. Food and Drug Administration and Drugs

Prescriptions

Prescription drugs are approved by the U.S. Food and Drug Administration (FDA) to be used on the order of a doctor. Prescription drugs have an indication or indications for use that the FDA approves. However, once a drug is approved for marketing, doctors can write a prescription for a purpose that is considered to be "off-label." Off-label use means that the drug is being prescribed for a reason other than the FDA-approved indication. This is perfectly legal and happens a lot. However, you as the patient should always be told whether you are being prescribed a drug for an off-label purpose. Your doctor should always tell you this information when the drug is prescribed for you.

OTC Drugs

OTC drugs are considered safe for consumers to use without a prescription. OTC containers contain information about drugs and proper use. However, I feel that the packaging is meant to grab your attention so you will buy the product. The information is there on how to use the product, but it can be hard to find and hard to read on the containers.

OTC PACKAGE LABELS

Figure 3-1 provides an example of what information is provided on OTC labels. As you can see, several types of information are provided on the containers (this information was obtained from several U.S. FDA websites and data information sources):

Drug Facts

Active Ingredient (in each tablet)   **Purpose**
Chlorpheniramine maleate 2 mg .... Antihistamine

Uses temporarily relieves these symptoms due to hay fever or other upper respiratory allergies: sneezing   ■ runny nose   ■ itchy, watery eyes   ■ itchy throat

Warnings
Ask a doctor before use if you have
■ glaucoma   ■ a breathing problem such as emphysema chronic bronchitis
■ trouble urinating due to an enlarged prostate gland

Ask a doctor or pharmacist before use if you are taking tranquilizers or sedatives

When using this product
■ drowsiness may occur   avoid alcoholic drinking
■ alcohol, sedatives, and tranquilizers may inrease drowsiness
■ be careful when driving a motor vehicle or operating machinery
■ excitablity may occur, especially in children

If pregnant or breast-feeding, ask a health professional before use.
Keep out of reach of children. In case of overdose, get medical help or contact a Poison Control Center right away.

Directions

adults and children 12 year and over	take 2 tablets every 4 to 6 hours: not more then 12 tablets in 24 hours
children 6 years to under 12 years	take 1 tablet every 4 to 6 hours: not more than 6 tablets in 24 hours
children under 6 years	ask a doctor ▼

Drug Facts   (continued)   ▲

Other Information ■ store at 20–25°C (68–77°) ■ protect from excessive moisture

Inactive Ingredients D&C yellow no. 10, lactose, magnesium stearate, microcrystalline cellulose, pregelatinized starch

---

Figure 3-1   Over-the-counter label example. (Source: U.S. Food and Drug Administration, www.fda.gov)

- Active ingredient: this is the active drug or drugs contained in the product
- Uses: what diseases or symptoms of diseases the drug is intended for
- Warnings:
  - When you should not use the product
  - Advice that you might need from your doctor before taking the drug
  - What some of the common side effects are with the drug
  - When you should stop taking the drug and call your doctor
  - If you are breastfeeding, contact your doctor before use
  - Keep the product out of reach of children
- Inactive ingredients: these might be colors or flavors added to the drug that do not have an effect on your symptoms or condition
- Purpose: what the drug is taken for, what condition or symptom it is meant to treat
- Directions:
  - How much to take
  - When to take it
  - How long you should take it for
  - What specific age categories the drug can be used for
- Other information:
  - How the drug should be stored
  - How much of certain ingredients the product contains, such as:
  –Sodium
  –Calcium
  –Potassium

TAMPER-RESISTANT PACKAGING FOR OTC DRUGS

The makers of OTC medicines use tamper-proof or tamper-evident packaging for their products (www.fda.gov/cder/consumerinfo/OTClabel.htm). Drugs with this packaging will generally have a plastic band around the top of the container that you tear off before you can open the package. Drug packages with this feature have a statement on the container describing how the package is tamper evident (www.fda.gov/cder/consumerinfo/OTClabel.htm).

AVAILABILITY OF DRUGS AS OTC DRUGS

Pharmaceutical companies submit applications to the FDA for new drugs. Drugs that are available as OTC drugs may have been listed as prescription drugs in the past. After a period of use, a company can petition the FDA to have a drug be made available without a prescription. Thus, the drug is now categorized as OTC, or a drug that can be bought without a prescription over the counter and can be sold at many different places.

Drugs to Treat Different Conditions

Drugs are available to treat many chronic conditions. There are many older and newer drugs that are available to treat conditions that, in the past, may have required a doctor's prescription for use. Your doctor writes prescriptions for medications based on several considerations. These factors include the history of your condition, side effects you might have had to similar medications, other health problems you have, and specific medication doses you might need to be treated successfully.

Although it is not always possible:

- Try to take as few drugs as possible
- Do not take multiple medications for the same condition
- If you are started on a new medication, can another drug that you take be stopped?
- Always check with your doctor before stopping any drug that you currently take!

Drugs Are Helpful and Have Been Used for Centuries

Drugs have the ability to ease suffering, help to control disease, and, in some cases, actually provide a cure for patients. Various types of drugs or medications have been ordered for patients for thousands of years. For centuries, drug therapies were mainly derived from plant sources. As a matter of fact, one of the most widely used drugs used to treat congestive heart failure is digoxin, a drug extracted from Digitalis lanata (foxglove) and used for centuries very successfully as the drug of choice for congestive heart failure. Please see Figure 3-2 for a photograph of a foxglove plant taken just outside of the town of Sawrey in the Cumbrian countryside in England.

Availability of Drugs

Drugs are available to treat many chronic conditions. There are many older and newer drugs that are available to treat conditions. Treating these conditions may include the use of prescription and OTC drugs. OTC drugs can be bought in many places in the United States: pharmacies, supermarkets, and convenience stores.

Monitor Yourself When You Take Drugs

With the ability to ease suffering comes the potential for drugs to also cause side effects, or adverse effects, or to provide no help whatsoever

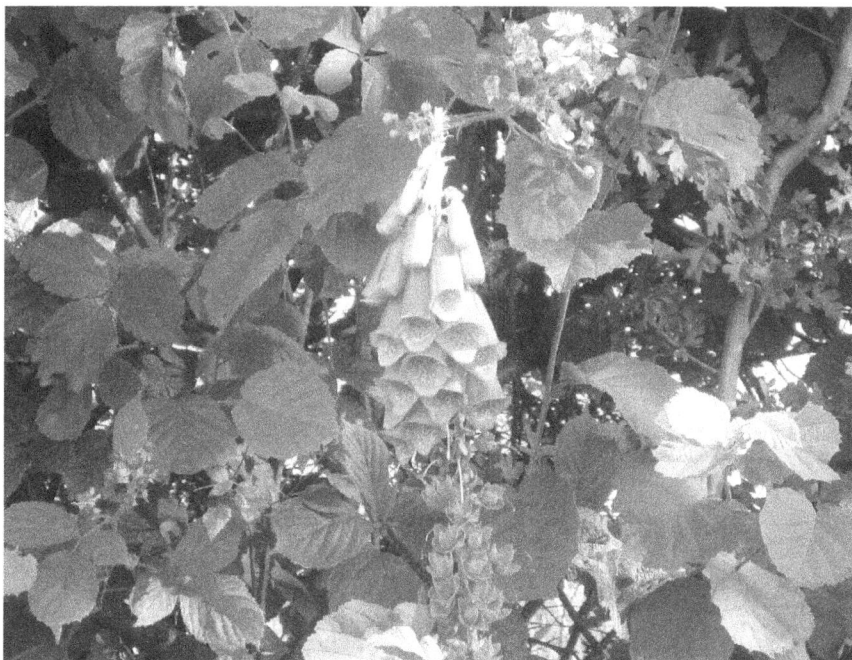

Figure 3-2   Foxglove plant.

for consumers. Side effects to medications are not only aggravating, but they are also a first warning indictor that something is wrong. Do not assume that when an adverse effect occurs that there is something that you are doing wrong or that it is your fault. You know your body better than anyone, so if something does not seem right and you are taking a medication (new or old), contact your physician or pharmacist. Always let them know what is happening with the drugs you take and the effects that they have on you.

Side effects, or adverse effects, to drug therapy are commonplace. If you experience a change in how you feel, a change in your bodily functions, or a dramatic decline in your functioning, contact your physician or pharmacist immediately. Side effects can occur with any medication, even those you may have taken for extended periods of time.

You will also need to monitor yourself when taking herbal and/or nutritional supplements. Many of these supplements have activity in the body that you might not be aware of, and because of this, you should always monitor yourself when taking them. Are you sick to your stomach when you take these products with other drugs that you take? Do the products make you drowsy or dizzy? Do these supplements affect other drugs that you need to take daily? Always ask what is in the supplements and what you might expect from the use of these products. If you purchase them on your own you may not have someone you can ask, so always let your pharmacist and doctor know what supplement you are taking. Take the containers with you when you see your doctor or pharmacist, let them examine the containers. Ask your health professionals what you need to know when taking these supplements.

WHAT YOU SHOULD KNOW ABOUT YOUR DRUGS

As noted in Chapter 2, you should always know the answers to the following questions about your drugs:

- What are the brand and generic names of the medications?
- What does it look like?

General Information about Drugs

- Why am I taking it?
- How much should I take, and how often?
- When is the best time to take it?
- How long will I need to take it?
- What side effects should I expect, and what should I do if they occur?
- What should I do if I miss a dose?
- Does this drug interact with my other medications or any foods?
- Does this drug replace anything else I was taking?
- Where and how do I store it?

BE AN ACTIVE PARTICIPANT IN YOUR HEALTH DECISIONS

Always work to participate in your health decision making, ask questions as needed, contact your doctor or pharmacist if you have questions, and continue to work with your doctors and pharmacists to help solve problems that may arise. You need not be embarrassed in asking questions and following up with your healthcare givers. You can help yourself by being knowledgeable about the medications prescribed for you or a loved one.

Summary

Medications may work for you as they should for a long period of time. Also be aware that drugs may not work as well as time goes by. They may also stop working altogether. If your drugs appear to not work any longer, your doctor may try another drug for you. There might also be another approach to help your conditions, such as diet, exercise, and so on. Always be patient with yourself during this process.

Be an active participant in your health and medication-taking decisions. Be as informed as you can be. This includes the decision you make to take medications.

CHAPTER FOUR

Understanding Drugs and Their Use

Introduction

The purpose of this chapter is to acquaint you with some general information about how drugs work. As I noted in Chapter 1, health professionals spend years studying drugs and their use. You as a patient are expected to take drugs as recommended by your doctor. After you read this chapter, you should know a little more about drugs and their use and purpose. Always be sure to check with your doctor or pharmacist if you have any questions about your drugs or how they will affect you. This chapter is meant to teach you more about drugs, but nothing in this chapter can replace the advice you receive from the health professionals (doctors, pharmacists, nurses, etc.) who provide care to you.

How Medications Work

Many of us do not like to take medications. But drugs allow us to live longer and better lives from a health standpoint. You, together with your doctor, can decide if the benefits of taking a drug will outweigh the risks that might be involved. Let's spend some time talking about how drugs work.

Dosage Forms

There are many different drug dosage forms. Medications can be:

- Pills (tablets)
- Capsules
- Liquids (like cough syrups)
- Injections (insulin, cancer chemotherapy drugs)
  - Into the veins
  - Into the muscle tissue
  - Under the skin (insulin for diabetes is injected just under the skin; insulin shot sites should be rotated from one body site to another to avoid dimpling of the skin)

There are also additional drug dosage forms that might be prescribed for you. For example, drugs can also be:

- Applied externally to the outside of the skin
  ○ Cream
  ○ Ointment
  ○ Transdermal patch (literally, across the skin)
    −A patch from which drugs are leached and enter the blood stream through the skin
- Taken under the tongue to be dissolved
- Inserted into the rectum (rectal suppositories are inserted into the rectum with gentle pushing)
- Inserted into the vagina for female medications (vaginal suppositories are inserted into the vagina with gentle pushing)
- Placed in the eye
  ○ Eye drops
  ○ Eye ointments
- Placed in the ear
  ○ Ear drops
- Placed under the tongue (sublingual tablets)
- Inhaled (sniffed) through the nose
- Inhaled through the mouth (breathed into the mouth)

Drugs for Chronic Conditions

There are many drugs that are used to treat chronic, or continuing, health conditions. These conditions may include high blood pressure, diabetes, heart failure, osteoporosis, or benign prostatic hypertrophy (BPH). A noncancerous condition of the male prostate gland is called BPH (swelling of the prostate). Your doctor can examine you to see whether you have BPH or prostate cancer.

Drugs for Acute Conditions

Other conditions are acute or short-term conditions. Some examples include viral or bacterial infections, coughs and colds, or skin conditions.

These conditions may require you to obtain prescriptions for various drug dosage forms.

Drugs to Treat Pain

There are many drugs to treat pain. They can include aspirin, acetaminophen (Tylenol), or ibuprofen (Advil, Nuprin). These drugs act on pain receptors at various parts of the body. There are also prescription pain medications that can include what are called narcotic analgesics. There are also drugs to treat arthritis that are available by prescription only.

Lock and Key Approach to Consider How Drugs Work

A lock and key approach can be helpful in depicting how drugs work in the body. Drugs are the keys, and the keys fit into locks in the body, causing an effect. Drugs may have agonist effects (the drug works by an active effect; e.g., it lowers high blood pressure or helps to reduce blood sugar levels) or antagonist effects (the drug works by stopping some action of the body). An antihistamine drug has an antagonist effect; it stops the effects of external objects (e.g., pollen, allergens, dust, etc.) that cause us to have an allergic reaction.

Examples of Actions of Drugs

Different drugs for high blood pressure act in different ways:

- Some drugs act directly in the brain
- Some drugs (β-blockers) act to block what are called β-receptors
- Some drugs are called calcium channel blockers

Drugs for high blood pressure can be likened to reducing pressure on a garden hose to decrease the pressure in the hose. Blood pressure drugs reduce the pressure in the blood stream by acting on the heart or the blood vessels. Antibiotics work by destroying bacteria either by breaking into the cells or by stopping the cells from reproducing. Antihistamines work by reducing the normal body reaction to pollen, allergens, weeds, plants, etc. Drugs also can act on the skin and penetrate into the blood stream or can be applied to the skin to stop an infection, rash, or skin eruption.

Herbs and Supplements Are Drugs Too

Also remember that the herbal and nutritional supplements that you take are drugs too. They may not be regulated like prescription and over-the-counter medications, but they also share the opportunity to bring you help or harm. Know what is in the supplements that you take, and be aware of their effect on how you feel and how you function. If you feel that something is just not right with how you feel, then it probably is not. Find out as much as you can about the supplements and what they can and cannot accomplish. Ask questions of your health providers to know how these supplements are or are not working. Be relentless in obtaining this information. If you cannot find someone who is knowledgeable about these nutritional supplements, seek help on your own from books, the Internet, or other health providers.

Cancer and Drugs

Cancer affects every family at one time or another. One of the major ways of treating many types of cancer is through the use of anticancer drugs. Drugs are taken to help reduce the size of tumors or to decrease the effect of cancer in the body. Treatments for cancer include surgery, radiation, and chemotherapy. Chemotherapy drugs can be tablets, capsules, or injected drugs.

Although the occurrence of cancer is devastating, there are more and more treatments available for people affected by cancer. As you can see in Figure 4-1, the number of new cancer drugs available is increasing each year. There are also many drugs that have already been approved for use that might be prescribed for you.

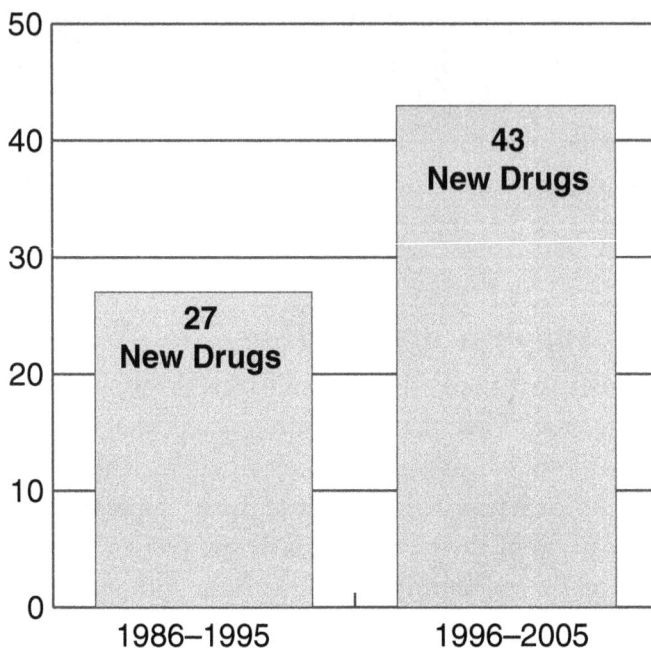

Figure 4-1   Cancer drug approval rates from 1986 to 2005. (Source: Bren L. Cancer drugs: Weighing the risks and benefits. *FDA Consumer Magazine,* **January/February 2007, available at http://www.fda.gov/fdac/features/2007/107_cancer.html; Accessed January 21, 2007.)**

Your doctor may want you to take multiple kinds of drugs to treat a cancer. This is common, and the drugs working in combination with one another work better than they might work by themselves. Cancer drugs work in several different ways. The drugs can kill the cancer cells and slow the growth of the tumor. The drugs can also counteract hormones that feed the cancer cells. Sometimes drugs that are male hormones will be used to treat a female cancer, and female hormones will be used to treat a male cancer.

What Men Need to Do before Taking a Drug for Prostate Problems

Men, do not hesitate in having your prostate checked annually or more frequently through prostate-specific antigen (PSA) blood work or through a digital rectal examination. Trust me, the digital examination of your rectum by a doctor using a plastic glove can help to catch any abnormality early, which is the best time to catch it!

Antianxiety Drugs

There are drugs called antianxiety agents that act on the central nervous system. One class of these drugs is benzodiazepines. This class of drugs is dangerous for seniors to take. If you take a drug in this class, make sure that you really need to take the drug. Please check with your doctor.

Drugs for Edema

Swelling in your feet or extremities is called edema. This build up of excess fluid can be treated by diuretics, which work to eliminate excess fluid from your body through actions on your kidneys. Edema can cause swelling of the feet. One of the symptoms of heart failure is edema. Another symptom is shortness of breath. Drugs called diuretics work on the kidneys to remove water from the body. Eliminating this fluid will help reduce edema (swelling) and also help lower blood pressure.

Side Effects

Many drugs have side effects. Always discuss how you are reacting to drugs with your doctor or pharmacist. It is not your fault if you experience a side effect.

Summary

Let you doctor know what you are experiencing when you take your drugs. Feel free to talk with your doctor, pharmacist, or nurse anytime about anything. The better the communication between you and your health providers is, the better the chances are that your health will improve.

Understanding Drugs and Their Use

CHAPTER FIVE

Dos and Don'ts of Drugs

Introduction

In this chapter, I will cover several things that you can do to help yourself with your drug taking. These tips are meant to explain actions that you "can do" with how you take your medications. Also, we will cover some things that you "should not do" when taking your medicines. Make sure that your doctor and pharmacist know all the medications that you are taking. These may be prescription, over-the-counter (OTC), or herbal products. Regardless of the type of medication, let your caregivers know all the drugs that you regularly take.

What to Do When You Are in Your Doctor's Office

Often when in physicians' offices, it is easy to be distracted and forget to ask questions that you feel are important. It might help if you do the following:

- Write down all your questions before you visit your doctor.
- Take this written sheet to the appointment with your doctor.
- Make a copy of the sheet, and provide the nurse that first sees you with the questions.
- Tell a loved one about your list and have them remind you of the items and what it is you wanted to ask.
- Write down all the drugs that you take, and make sure the doctor sees this list.
- Have someone go to the appointment with you.
- Follow up after the appointment to ensure that you have remembered all of the questions and have the answers that you need.
- Keep asking if you did not receive the answers that you need to understand treatments, therapies, drugs, etc.
- When you see a physician or pharmacist, you are the most important person in the encounter, so make sure you find out what you need to know.

Don't Leave the Pharmacy without These!

The Institute for Safe Medication Practices (ISMP) suggests that you know about the drugs you are prescribed before leaving the pharmacy. The ISMP is a 10-year-old nonprofit organization working to make the medication use process less prone to errors and mistakes. Make sure that you know the answers to the following questions before you take your medications.

"Before you leave the pharmacy, your pharmacist should give you printed information about the medication and make sure that you understand the answers to these questions:

- What are the brand and generic names of the medications?
- What does it look like?
- Why am I taking it?
- How much should I take, and how often?
- When is the best time to take it?
- How long will I need to take it?
- What side effects should I expect, and what should I do if they happen?
- What should I do if I miss a dose?
- Does this interact with my other medications or any foods?
- Does this replace anything else I was taking?
- Where and how do I store it?" (ISMP, 2007)

What to Do to Help Your Drug Taking

Let's examine what you can do to help your medicine taking. I recommend that you use one pharmacy for your prescriptions. In this way, all your records for taking your prescriptions can be kept in one spot. If at all possible, try to improve your health by other means besides taking prescriptions. This will not always be possible; you may need to take medicines for several conditions. If your doctor can write your prescriptions so that you only need to take your drugs once a day or if your medicine taking can be simplified, you have a better chance of complying with your medicines. Also, do not take multiple medicines for the same condition unless you have been told to do so by your doctor.

Brown Bag Reviews

One of the best things that you can do at least once a year is to take all your medicines to your doctor so that you can let your doctor see what drugs you are taking. I encourage you to do this with your pharmacist as well. Set up a time that is convenient for both you and your caregivers. This allows them to examine all the drugs that you are taking.

Take as Few Drugs as Possible

Always try to take as few medications as possible. When starting a new therapy, find out how long you will need to take it. Also, determine whether you can stop other medications because of the new therapy. Never hesitate in asking for help with the questions and problems that you have with your medication therapies.

If you take eight or more drugs, ask your doctor whether there is a way to eliminate a drug or two that you simply do not need to continue to take. See Figure 5-1 for a diagram showing what you can do to possibly take fewer medications.

Improve Your Medicine Taking

There are several things that you can do to improve your medicine taking. I call it "connect the dots." See Figure 5-2 for tips to help you with your drug-taking needs. I use this diagram to indicate several things that you can do to lessen problems that you might have with drugs. With your doctor's approval, stop taking drugs that may be dangerous for you to continue to take. When at all possible, do not take several drugs for the same ailment. If you can have drugs that you take just once a

When at all possible – take fewer medications

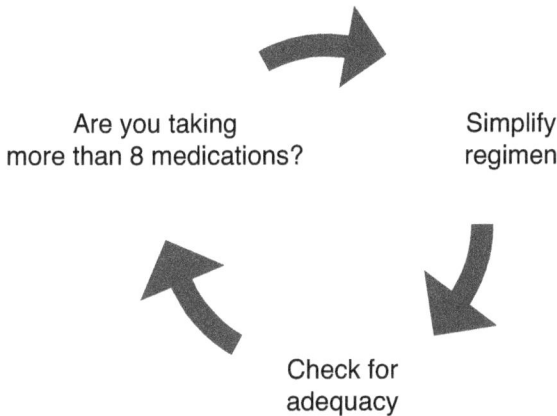

Are you taking more than 8 medications?

Simplify regimen

Check for adequacy

Figure 5-1   What to do to take fewer medications.

day, your compliance with the drugs will improve. Follow a daily routine when taking your drugs. Working with your doctors and pharmacist, find the best time for you to take your drugs each day. This may be in the morning, with breakfast or lunch, or at another time. If you can avoid taking drugs, you will probably be better off. Always check with your doctor before you start or stop taking a drug or drugs.

Know who your pharmacist is, and find a pharmacist that you can trust. Ask your doctor and pharmacist for advice on how best to throw out old or outdated (not fresh anymore) drugs. You will, from time to time, accumulate extra doses of prescription drugs, bottles with one or two tablets or capsules in them, ointment or cream tubes with small amounts left in them, etc. The leftover medications may be outdated or simply extra doses that were not taken. The normal inclination is to save these medications for potential future use. I do not suggest doing this; some medications such as antibiotics should be discarded after use and the correct period of dosing in the therapy. It can be confusing to try to manage the many small amounts that are left over after a time.

Discontinue dangerous drugs

Do not take multiple
medications for same condition

Once daily drugs

Follow a routine for
taking medications

Non-drug alternatives

Know your pharmacist ⟶ Discard old and
outdated drugs

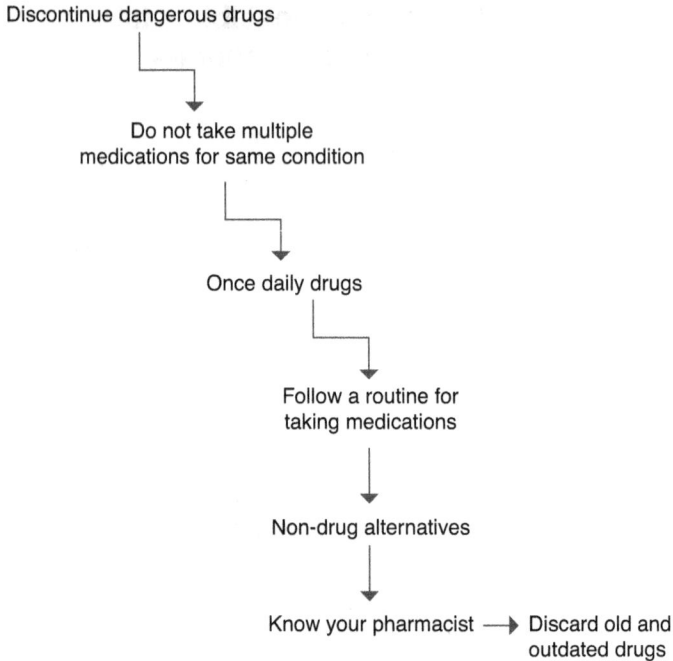

Figure 5-2   Connect the dots!

When filled, most prescriptions require that the expiration date for the medication be listed on the prescription label. Make sure your pharmacist tells you where to look for this date. I would suggest that you either take the drugs back to your pharmacist for disposal or find out whether there is a place in your community where you can take the drugs for proper disposal. I would not suggest that you flush them down a toilet or garbage disposal. Be very cautious about dumping them in with your normal garbage. It is too easily accessible to pets. Boehringer (2004) suggests the following if you use the garbage to throw out your medications:

- Keep all medicines in their original container with childproof lids attached.
- Mark out anyone's name that may be printed on a prescription container.
- Place liquid in a plastic sealable bag in case it leaks or breaks.
- Put everything inside a sturdy container (like a plain brown box).

- Add a nontoxic but bad-tasting product like cayenne pepper to the container.
- Make this container the last thing you put in the garbage can before pickup.

Don't Accept Directions Such as "Take as Directed"

There are some things that you need to know about your drugs. Always ask your pharmacist and doctor for help with any questions about your medications. Never accept directions such as "Take as directed" or "As directed" on your prescriptions. Your physician and pharmacist need to explain in detail how you are to take any medicine. Keep asking until you receive proper directions.

Adverse Effects

Sometimes adverse drug effects do not occur with the first use of the drug by a patient. Instead, a drug's adverse effect may be additive and may not occur until after multiple uses of the drug or perhaps after many years of use. Also, a drug by itself may not lead to an adverse drug event, but the combination of the drug plus a new additional medication or medications may lead to an adverse drug event. Often, drugs will have a side effect. Sometimes these effects can be lessened by taking the drugs with food or at different times of the day. Always ask your doctor and pharmacist for advice on when best to take your medicines.

PREDICTABLE SIDE EFFECTS

Some drugs lead to very predictable side effects that are not worrisome. For example, some drugs cause the urine, sweat, sputum, saliva, or tears to be colored (red-orange in the case of rifampin [Rifadin]) or darker in color (yellow in the case of B vitamins or red-orange in the case of phenazopyridine [AZO Standard, URISTAT], a urinary tract analgesic taken orally). These discolorations are nothing to be alarmed about and are harmless. In fact, they may indicate that you have been taking the medication in question.

Some coloration that might appear in your body fluid wastes is not normal and is a warning sign that something is wrong. For example, if you notice blood specs in your urine or feces, this is not normal, and you should be concerned and alert your care providers. Also, if you are unable to urinate or defecate or are having trouble doing so (more than usual), this is a cause for concern, and you should alert your physician and pharmacist. Some drugs may have this affect on patients, but it is always a good idea to check and make sure that others know of your troubles in this regard. If you notice blood in the stool, this is always a cause for concern. This may be due to a mild (hemorrhoids) or serious condition (colon cancer). Regardless, you need to view this symptom seriously and check to find out what is causing the symptom.

If Your Drugs Do Not Work, It Is Not Your Fault

There are times when a drug that you are prescribed may not work as you or your physician expects. This is not your fault, and you should not feel that you are somehow to blame. In these cases, you may need to be placed on a different medication. Also, there are instances when a drug may lose its ability to be effective over time in patients. There is great variability in how a drug will work in general, and there is certainly a difference in drug activity from patient to patient. Be patient with yourself as you work with your care providers to find the best drug for you with the optimum ability to provide you with the help that you need.

Risks and Benefits of Drugs

All drugs have risks and benefits associated with use. Some drugs that may be risky may also be drugs that you must take for your ailments. Please do not start or stop taking a drug without first checking with your doctor. Your pharmacist can also answer questions that you might have about the drugs that you take. Even some drugs commonly taken for pain relief need to be taken with caution. You can feel safe taking drugs like acetaminophen for pain relief. Just be sure to take the recommended amount or a smaller amount to take care of the pain that you might have. Other drugs like ibuprofen or aspirin can be hard on your stomach. Take these drugs with a snack, such as a cookie or cracker, to lessen their impact on your stomach. There are prescription drugs for arthritis that you should only take as a last resort when other drugs have not worked for you.

One side effect of some drugs that you may take may be depression. You may not expect this to happen. If you notice any changes in how you feel or how you feel about yourself when you start taking a new medicine or even after you have taken the drug for awhile, let your doctor know how you are feeling (Fincham, 2005).

Don't Use Imported Drugs

I urge you not to obtain drugs from foreign sources. There are just too many questions about these drugs and their proper use. I cannot urge you strongly enough to be very cautious about the drugs that you obtain from foreign sources. The quality of many of these substances is suspect. I suggest that you do not use imported drugs from either Mexico or Canada.

Advisory Labels on Prescription Bottles

When we have prescriptions filled, sometimes they will have advisory or warning labels attached to them. Ask your pharmacist about these labels if they do not make sense to you. This label indicates that you should not take the medicine with any alcoholic beverage (wine, beer, or whisky). Don't be offended if these labels are on your bottles and you don't drink. Your pharmacist is trying to help you avoid a bad outcome in case the drugs that you take would interact badly with other things that you might consume.

Dos and Don'ts of Drugs

When to Take Your Medicines

Not only is it difficult to take your medications in and of itself, but often, there are requirements to take your medicine with food, without food, at meals, or at some other time that may be difficult to remember. It is always good to ask your pharmacist about which of your medications are affected or unaffected by food intake. The pharmacist will have reference materials that can help you to learn which of your medications are best taken with food or without food.

Some medications need to be taken with food in order to be absorbed from the stomach. One such drug is nitrofurantoin (Macrodantin). Some medications have caustic effects on the stomach if taken without food, and thus, your doctor may want you to take the drug with food to minimize your chances of stomach upset. Other drugs are absorbed whether or not you take them with food, so again, to minimize stomach upset, you may want to take them with food. Medications that should be taken with food have increased rates of absorption and higher blood levels when taken with food. Also remember that taking your drugs with food does not mean that you have to eat a five-course meal in order to take your medications. It may be as simple as taking your medications with a soda cracker, piece of bread, or glass of milk. It is not the quantity of food that is important; instead, it is just a matter of having something in your stomach to help the medication either work better or cause less stomach upset. Some drugs you will need to always take on an empty stomach. Some medications are made inactive by consumption with food. Always check with your pharmacist for clarification about when to take your drugs.

Forgetting Doses and What to Do about It

What if you forget a dose? The normal inclination is to go ahead and take it right away. This is not always the best course of action. Let me go through some specific examples of when and when not to take the forgotten dose.

Once-a-day drugs can be a beneficial way for you to improve your medication compliance. If you take a drug once daily in the morning, but you forget the dose and remember you forgot it early in the afternoon or evening, go ahead and take the medication the same day. Then resume the normal dosing time the next day. If it is almost time to take your next dose, do not double up. If you forget about the dosing until the next day, do not double up on the dose when you take the dose the next day. There are exceptions, and it is always best to check with your physician to make sure how you should best handle skipped doses.

Some drugs may need to be taken twice a day or more. If you take a medication twice daily and forget to take the dose at one point of the day and if it is fairly close to the dosing time, you can go ahead and take it, spacing the dose as far as you can from the next dose administration. Do not arbitrarily double or triple the dose if you forget several doses and do not remember when you took the last dose. In this case, ask your physician for advice. If you are taking an antibiotic and forget to take a dose, take it as soon as you can remember to do so, and then resume the normal schedule as soon as you can.

Do whatever you can to take your medications as prescribed. If there are specific ways that you have been told to take your drugs, always ask your doctor or pharmacist for tips and advice on ways that can help you be more compliant. You should not be embarrassed by asking questions and following up with your healthcare providers. You can help yourself do better by being knowledgeable about the medications prescribed for you or a loved one.

Special Handling of Some Drugs

Various medications may require special handling, storage, or administration techniques. This chapter presents a listing of some issues to consider with certain dosage forms that may require you to do different things regarding their use. Some medications require refrigeration before and during their use. Some drugs for injection supplied in a multiuse container are meant to be refrigerated. Other medications may be stored in a refrigerator, but it is not necessary to do so. An example is insulin for injection. Insulin bottles are stored in a refrigerated environment to protect their shelf life (or freshness period). However, the insulin in these containers after they are opened does not need to be refrigerated but just stored at room temperature. Most people continue to refrigerate their insulin bottles, but it is not necessary. If you are traveling, you should keep the insulin in an environment where the bottle(s) will not become excessively heated. You can also purchase insulin on trips in pharmacies as you go along. You do not necessarily need to stock up in advance and try to arrange refrigeration for the insulin.

To Refrigerate or Not to Refrigerate— That Is the Question

Some of your medications (tablets, capsules) do not need to be refrigerated. Some people feel that keeping their medications in the refrigerator will assure that they stay fresh. This is not the case; in fact, the moisture and humidity present in the refrigerator may actually be bad for the medications. The moisture will affect the stability of many tablets and capsules. In fact, all prescription medications coming from the manufacturer contain either a sodium silicate contained in a semiporous packet or small canister that absorbs excess moisture in the container. Again, this is because the tablets and capsules need to be stored in a moisture-free environment. These sodium silicate packets are harmful if swallowed, so please do not ingest them or have them within reach of a child or a pet.

Other liquid preparations, such as cough syrups and pain relief liquids, *do not* need to be refrigerated. Some antibiotic prescriptions (e.g., sulfamethoxazole/trimethoprim [Bactrim]) also *do not* need to be refrigerated.

Creams and Ointments

Creams and ointments are required to have expiration dating; the expiration date for creams and ointments can be found impressed on the bottom "crimp" of the ointment or cream tube. It may be difficult to read, but with a magnifying glass, you can spot the date. Again, if you cannot see where it is, ask your pharmacist to guide you to the spot. I do not get as excited about using external ointment and cream medications at a point after their initial use and before their expiration dates. They should never be used past the expiration date that is on the actual tube itself, but if the salve is for an infection, and the infection reoccurs at a point in the future, I see nothing wrong with saving the product and using the external cream or ointment in the future. Eye drops are an exception to this. I would not use the eye drops in a container after 90 days of initially opening the container because the sterility of the contents of the product meant for instilling in the eye simply cannot be guaranteed after the product is opened. I would not save eye drops for future use.

Easy-Open Containers

If you cannot open a container or access your medications, ask your pharmacist or physician for alternate containers or drugs that you can access. Please do not feel that you are the only one who has trouble opening and accessing medication containers; it is common, and you are not unique in having this trouble.

Don't Share Your Drugs with Others

It is not a good idea to share your medications with others. You simply do not have all of the information that you need to adequately decide on diagnoses, dosage forms, or whether or not someone else is allergic to a medication. Also, it is not a good idea to be the recipient of someone else's offer to help you out by sharing their medication with you.

Dos and Don'ts of Drugs

Crushing or Splitting Your Tablets

Certain medications should not be crushed or split. Some products may have a very unpleasant taste unless they are coated and thus are not meant to be split. Other medications may irritate the skin or mucous membranes if split open. Products that are meant to be dissolved over a longer period of time should not be crushed or split. For example, if a tablet is a controlled-release product taken once or twice daily, it should not be crushed or split. The material in the tablet or capsule is coated such that it is slowly released over a period of time. Enteric-coated tablets are meant to be dissolved in the intestines and not in the upper stomach. As was previously noted, these enteric, controlled-release, and/or extended-release medications should not be crushed or split open. Always check with your pharmacist before you try to split a tablet.

Some tablets are meant to be dissolved under the tongue. These so-called sublingual tablets (literally translated "under the tongue") should not be split in half either. Other tablets referred to as buccal tablets are meant to dissolve in the side of the mouth and should not be split or cut in any manner.

For the most part, capsules should not be split in half or otherwise opened so as to split the dosage amount. There are some products that are available as capsules that can be opened; your pharmacist will be able to provide you with information about specific capsule products that can or cannot be opened. Other capsules called liquid gels (or perhaps another name) contain liquid medication and should not be split open. The names of these types of dosage forms include perle (e.g., benzonatate [Tessalon Perles]), gel cap, soft capsule formulation, and others. Always check with your pharmacist if you have questions about whether a capsule can be opened or not. Your physician may not always know what formulations are available, so your pharmacist is always the best source of information. If your pharmacist has a question, they can always call the physician to clarify the dose and dosage form that you need.

Other medications may not be stable unless they are in the original dosage form, or they simply cannot be split open. An example of a tablet that cannot be split open is sildenafil (Viagra) 100-mg tablets; it is not possible to split this tablet into two 50-mg tablets without an uneven break of the tablet.

Some tablets have a definite recessed mark on the top of the tablet and can be split in half. This can be done either by using your fingers to split the tablet or by placing the tablet on a plate and using a table knife to gently pry the tablet in two. If you are unsure how to do this, ask your pharmacist for assistance or have a family member help you with this task. Use caution when splitting these tablets; do not use excessive force or have your hand or fingers under the tablet that you are trying to cut in half with an instrument.

Don't Use Outdated Drugs!

Outdated drugs should never be used for any purpose. Drugs are expensive, but using drugs past an expiration date is risky business and not recommended. Even though the tablet or capsule may appear to be new and shows no apparent signs of decay, the drug must not be used. Drugs for heart ailments, such as β-blockers, angiotensin-converting enzyme (ACE) inhibitors, and nitroglycerin tablets, are examples of drugs with a narrow therapeutic range, and any deviance from normal levels obtained with fresh drugs can be life threatening. The level of the drug in the blood must be within a very narrow range in order for it to be effective.

In other instances, use of outdated drugs may not only cause no therapeutic effect, but it can also be life threatening due to outdated drug breakdown products contained in the dosage form. The use of outdated tetracycline antibiotics can be used as an example. Outdated tetracyclines should never be administered. The breakdown products of outdated tetracycline products are highly toxic to the kidneys (nephrotoxic) and have, on occasion, produced a kidney disease termed Fanconi-like syndrome.

Use a Proper Measuring Device for Liquid Medications

Never use a measuring cup to measure medication that comes in drop form. This could lead to a very large overdose with toxic effects.

Expense of Drugs

Prescriptions are expensive and becoming more so each year. Do what you can to obtain help paying for your medications before you skip doses in order to save money. Do not feel badly if you cannot afford your medications; you are not alone. A recent study found that two thirds of seniors do not let their physicians or nurses know that they cannot afford their medications. In defense of patients, most physicians do not know how much medications cost and thus are buffered from the burdens their patients experience in trying to afford the cost of drugs.

Be Your Own Best Advocate

You need to be your own best advocate when it comes to receiving your healthcare services. Your caregivers should take the time to answer your questions and help you to understand what you should do with medicines or your health conditions. The first rule in medicine is to do no harm. Second, if your drugs are working okay for you, don't try to fix something that is not broken. Finally, ask your doctor if there are different ways for you to "fix" your drug regimens.

Make Taking Medicine Part of Your Daily Routine

Try to make taking your medicine a very routine part of your day. This might mean that you take your drugs in the morning around the time you eat breakfast. You might want to take your drugs just after you brush your teeth or at another remembrable time. You might also find it easier to be compliant with your medicines if you take them before you go to bed in the evening. Also, try to make a note of what you have taken and when you took it.

Summary

Finally, here is a list of summary items for you to consider. Always know why you are taking your medicines. What are they used for? What are their names? What do I do if I skip a dose or forget to take it? When should I take my medicines? Should I take them with food or a snack or on an empty stomach? Finally, where should I store my medicines? Steel medicine cabinets in your bathroom are not a good choice for storing your medicines. They trap moisture and heat and can lead to deterioration of your medicines. Find a place to store your medicines that is away from heat, light, and moisture. Find the most convenient place for you to help you remember to take your medicines.

Participate in your health decision making, ask questions as needed, contact your doctor or pharmacist if you have questions, and continue to work with your doctors and pharmacists to help solve problems that may arise. Medications may work for you as they should for a long period of time. Also be aware that drugs may not work as well as time goes by. They may also stop working altogether.

See Figure 5-3 for a summary of things that can do to help yourself with your medicine taking. These include:

- Use one pharmacy for your prescriptions
- Use nondrug alternatives if possible
- Ask your doctor to write prescriptions in such a manner that simplifies your drug taking
- Reduce or eliminate taking multiple medications for the same condition

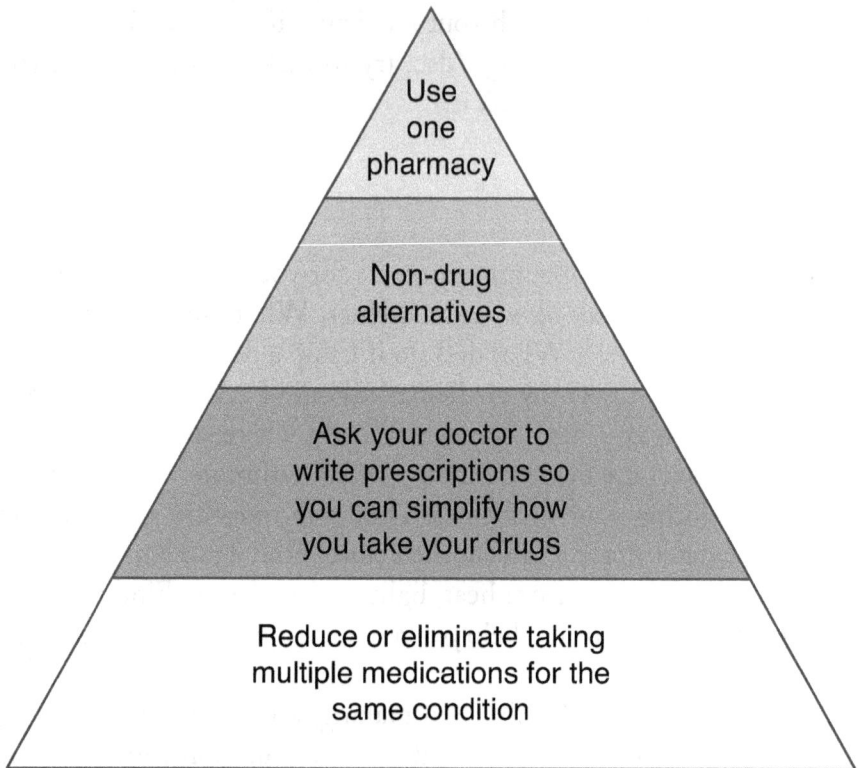

Figure 5-3   Pyramid for successful dos and don'ts with medicines.

References

Boehringer SK. What's the best way to dispose of medications? *Pharmacist's Letter* 2004;20(200415).

Fincham J. Drugs that cause depression. *Bottom Line Health*, June 2005.

Institute for Safe Medication Practices (ISMP). Key questions. Available at http://www.ismp.org/Newsletters/consumer/alerts/Brochure.asp; accessed March 15, 2007.

CHAPTER SIX

Tips to Enhance Compliance with Your Medications

Introduction

This chapter will provide you with information about patient compliance with medications. You will also be provided with some tips to help you be compliant and have better health. Do not feel that you are the only one that struggles with taking your medicine. Many of us do!

Hey, This Is Not Easy!

Taking medicines can be difficult. It is both hard to remember when to take your drugs and difficult to remember if you have forgotten to take your medicines. You may have several diseases and feel poorly. If you have several diseases, you are likely taking several prescriptions, at least one medicine per disease. To make things more complicated, you may have to take the different drugs several times a day or at different times.

Effects of Noncompliance

The results of noncompliance are devastating. Seniors are often readmitted to hospitals with drug-related problems within 6 months of initial discharge from hospitals. Drug-related noncompliance is a major reason for the need to readmit seniors for further care.

Drug Expense

Prescriptions are expensive and becoming more so each year. Do what you can to obtain help paying for your medications before you skip doses in order to save money. Drugs are expensive and becoming more expensive every year. But if you do not take your medications you may pay for additional healthcare expenses. By not complying with medications, you may need to pay for more drugs, physician visits, emergency room visits, and/or hospitalizations.

Types of Compliance

One way to examine medicine taking and classify several types of compliance behavior is depicted in Figure 6-1, and the segments are explained here:

- *Initial compliance*—Having your prescription filled initially at a pharmacy. Approximately 10% of all new prescriptions are never filled by patients.
- *Partial compliance*—Taking some of your medication as prescribed. The rate of noncompliance is 50% across all drug types and types of patients.
- *Total compliance*—Taking your medications exactly as prescribed. Some of you are perfect! You take all your drugs all the time.
- *Hypercompliance*—Taking too much of your medication. This can be really dangerous. Never exceed the dosage your doctor prescribes.

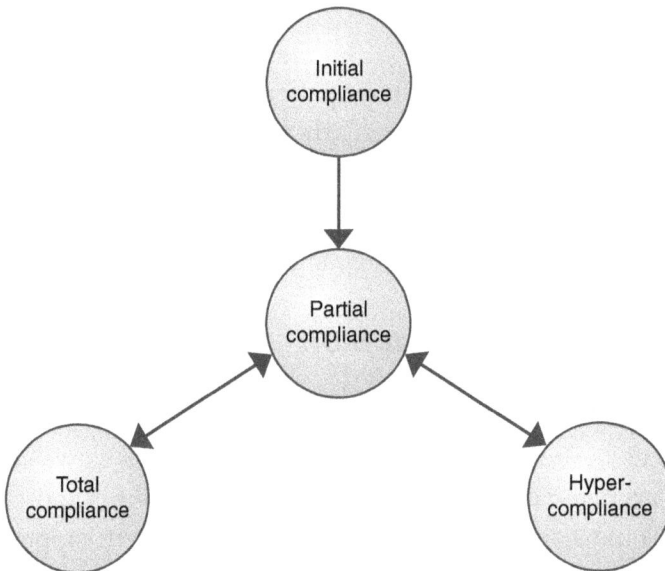

Figure 6-1   Types of compliance. (Source: Fincham JE. Patient Compliance with Medications: Issues and Opportunities. Binghamton, NY: Pharmaceutical Products Press, 2007, p. 80.)

What Factors Influence Compliance?

Several factors may make it hard for you to take your medicines correctly 100% of the time. These factors include:

- Living by yourself
- Having several diseases
- Taking several drugs
- Taking the medicine is very complicated
- Not feeling good

If you live by yourself, it may be hard to do things alone, including taking your medicines. If you have several diseases, it may be hard to keep track of what you are supposed to do for each ailment. Taking several drugs makes things more complicated. Also, the way that you are to take the drugs may be hard to control and maintain. In addition to all of this, you just may not feel very good, and this will make taking your drugs difficult.

Have others help to improve your patient compliance. Having someone call, e-mail, or visit you regularly to remind you to be compliant might be just what you need. If this becomes a routine contact for you, you may be helped a great deal along the path to better compliance.

Noncompliance Is Common

Rates of Compliance

Many of us have trouble with taking our medicines as we should. In fact, the average rate of correct drug taking behavior is approximately 50%. This means that, on average, we do what we are supposed to do with our drugs correctly half of the time. As I said before, if you have some difficulty, you are not alone! Do not feel badly if this is what happens to you. Make a decision to try to do better and improve your compliance

Importance of Information and Communication

There are things that happen because your doctor does not provide clear information either to you or your pharmacist. The directions for how you are to take your medicine may be unclear. You may not know how many times you should have your prescriptions refilled. The amount that you are to take is not clear to you. Or you may be confused by the names or strengths of the drugs that you are to take.

Sometimes you receive information from so many sources that you become confused. This is common and happens to many people. Also, the material that you are provided may be unreliable. This is why it is important to have credible sources of information. Your doctor and your pharmacist can help you to find the right information to meet your needs.

Aids to Help You Be More Compliant

There are several types of aids to help you improve your compliance. They include:

- Calendars
- Diaries
- Packaging
  - Divided pill containers
  - Non–child-resistant closures
- Electronic monitors
- Special packaging
- Social support
- Making compliance routine

Using a calendar means just indicating on a wall calendar or other type of calendar when you have taken your medicine or need to take your medicine doses. Diaries are a book or other type of journal where you write down when you have taken your medicines, how you feel when you take the drug, and whether you are experiencing any adverse effects. Having your pharmacist provide you with a bottle that you can open easily helps you take your drugs too. You can ask your pharmacist to dispense prescriptions to you in non–child-resistant packages.

Sophisticated but Helpful Devices to Aid Compliance

One of the simple yet sophisticated compliance packaging programs is depicted in Figure 6-2. This photograph shows the Medicine-On-Time system. This particular system color codes the time of day you are to take your medicines and packages them together in a sealed pack-

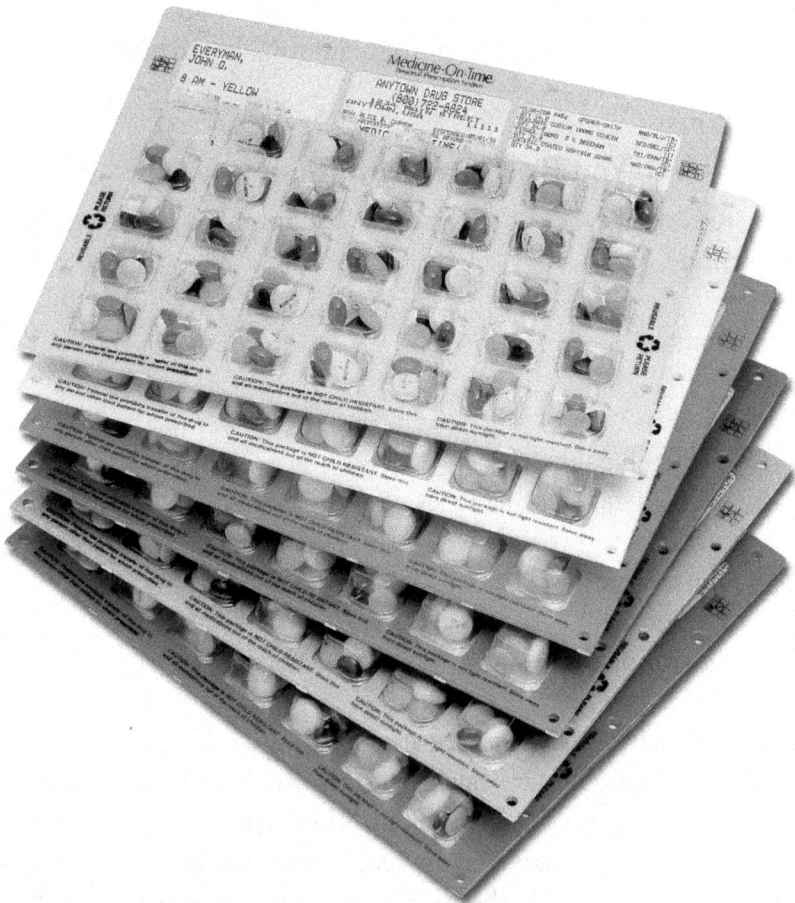

Figure 6-2   The Medicine-On-Time system. (Source: Medicine-On-Time © 2004, used with permission.)

age that you take the contents of when you are supposed to. See Figure 6-3 for a picture of what these individual packaged doses look like when packaged.

There are also more sophisticated types of compliance aids. See Figure 6-4 for a picture of compliance watch. The compliance watch is a Medicine-On-Time system device that provides patients with a wrist-watch reminder of the times and drugs to take during the day. There are other devices that might include electronic monitors or special packaging to help you be compliant. Having a family member or friend provide support can help you remember to be compliant too. This might be simply having someone call you to tell you to take your drugs.

Make Compliance with Your Drugs Routine

Make compliance and taking your medicine a routine part of your day. Take your drugs at the same time each day, and get in the habit of being compliant and having a set time to take your doses. Through providing you better communication and clear directions, your care-givers can make it easier for you to be compliant. Your pharmacist may be able to use different types of packages other than a tablet vial that will allow you to visually see what you need to take. Also, you can see the doses that you missed taking.

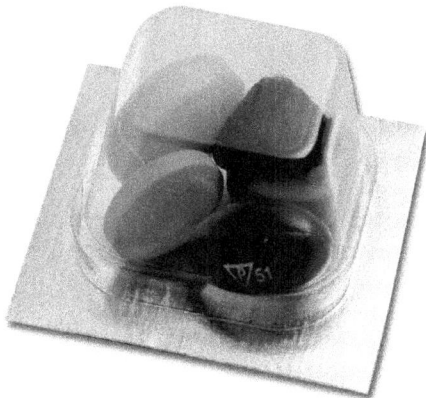

Figure 6-3   A sample of an individual packaged dose from the Medicine-On-Time system. (Source: Medicine-On-Time © 2004, used with permission.)

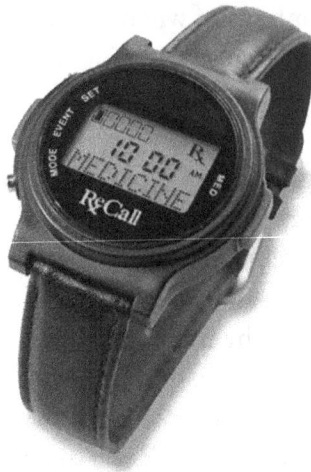

Figure 6-4   The compliance watch is a Medicine-On-Time system device that provides patients with a wristwatch reminder of the times and drugs to take during the day. (Source: Medicine-On-Time © 2004, used with permission.)

What Do You Do if You Forget a Dose?

What do you do if you miss a dose? If you take a drug once daily in the morning and forget the dose, but remember you forgot it early in the afternoon or evening, go ahead and take the medication the same day. Then resume the normal dosing time the next day. If it is almost time to take your next dose, do not double up. If you forget about the dosing until the next day, do not double up on the dose when you take the dose the next day. There are exceptions, and it is always best to check with your physician about how to best handle skipped doses.

If you take a medication twice daily and forget to take the dose at one point in the day and if it is fairly close to the dosing time, you can go ahead and take it, spacing the dose as far as you can from the next dose administration. Do not arbitrarily double or triple the dose if you forget several doses or do not remember when you took the last dose. In this case, ask your physician for advice. If you are taking an antibiotic and you forget to take a dose, take it as soon as you can remember to do so, and then resume the normal schedule as soon as possible.

Do Your Best!

Do whatever you can to take your medications as prescribed. If there are specific ways that you have been told to take your drugs, always ask for tips and advice on ways that can be helpful to you in complying. Most of us take more than one medication; more than 60% of office visits to physicians result in one or more prescriptions being written. This makes our task complicated. If we are to take medications in a special manner, this can hinder our best efforts to be compliant. That is why advice can be helpful from your physician, pharmacist, family members, friends, or acquaintances.

When to Take Your Drugs: With or Without Food

Not only is it difficult to take your medications in and of itself, but often, there are requirements to take your medicine with food, without food, at meals, or at some other time that may be difficult to remember. It is always good to ask your pharmacist about which of your medications are affected or unaffected by food intake. The pharmacist will have reference materials that can help you to learn which of your medications are best taken with food or without food.

Some medications need to be taken with food in order to be absorbed from the stomach. Some medications have caustic effects on the stomach if taken without food, and thus, your doctor may want you to take the drug with food to minimize your chances of stomach upset. Other drugs are absorbed whether or not you take them with food, so again, to minimize stomach upset, you may want to take them with food. Medications that should be taken with food have increased rates of absorption and higher blood levels when taken with food.

Other medications are made inactive by consumption with food; for example, tetracycline (Sumycin) is inactivated by taking it with food. Some medications should not be taken with food or food byproducts that contain certain substance, such as calcium.

Stopping Your Drugs for a Reason

There are occasions when you should stop taking your medications and await further advice from your caregivers. This is intelligent non-compliance. You may be advised to stop taking the medication altogether, another medication may be prescribed for you, or you may be asked to be seen by a physician. In other cases, because of side effects that are occurring, you may be advised to stop taking your medication and be seen by your doctor.

In some cases, by monitoring your condition or symptoms, it may not be necessary for you to continue to take medications. Some drugs are prescribed on an as-needed basis. An examples of this might be oral antihistamines that are taken for allergies that may vary during the year; thus, they may not need to be taken year round. In another instance, the dose of a drug, such as insulin to treat diabetes, may require that you alter the amount injected or the amount injected automatically by an insulin pump.

Also, you may need to alter how you take a drug, such as digoxin (Lanoxin) to treat congestive heart failure, if your pulse falls below a certain minimum amount. If your pulse is less than 65, many doctors do not want the dose taken that day. This is something for your doctor to change.

Adverse Drug Effects

Virtually every drug used has the potential for an adverse effect or side effect. What is the difference? Well, an adverse effect is always a negative outcome, whereas a side effect may or may not be negative. It is important to monitor your body functions to monitor for effects that are normal for you.

If you notice a change in how you feel or a difference in your body functions, you may be experiencing an adverse drug reaction. Contact your physician and your pharmacist and explain your current symptoms and the drugs that you are taking. As noted, some drugs lead to very predictable side effects that are not worrisome. For example, some drugs cause the urine, sweat, sputum, saliva, or tears to be colored (red-orange in the case of rifampin [Rifadin]) or darker in color (yellow in the case of B vitamins or red-orange in the case of phenazopyridine [AZO Standard, URISTAT], a urinary tract analgesic taken orally). These discolorations are nothing to be alarmed about and are harmless.

Some coloration that might appear in your body fluid wastes is not normal and is a warning sign that something is wrong. For example, if you notice blood specs in your urine or feces, this is not normal, and you should be concerned and alert your care providers. Also, if you are unable to urinate or defecate or are having trouble doing so (more than usual), this is a cause for concern, and you should alert your physician and pharmacist. Some drugs may have this affect on patients, but it is always a good idea to check and make sure that others know of your troubles in this regard.

Sometimes adverse drug effects do not occur with the first use of the drug by a patient. Instead, a drug's adverse effect may be additive and may not occur until after multiple uses of the drug or perhaps after many years of use. Also, a drug by itself may not lead to an adverse drug event, but the combination of the drug plus a new additional medication or medications may lead to an adverse drug event.

Considerations for You to Think About

Lack of Therapeutic Effects

There are times when a drug that you are prescribed may not work as you or your physician expects. This is not your fault, and you should not feel that you are somehow to blame. In these cases, you may need to be placed on a different medication. Also, there are times when a drug may lose its ability to be effective over time with patients. There is great variability in how a drug will work in general, and there is certainly a difference in drug activity from patient to patient. Be patient with yourself as you work with your care providers to find the best drug for you with the optimum ability to provide you with the help that you need.

Drug-Free Improvement

Also, you may find that you can feel better without taking anything or by discontinuing a certain medication. This is great, but just make sure that you and your physician(s) are all on the same page when it comes to discontinuing the drugs that you are taking. There are many drugs that are meant to be taken for a short period of time anyway. Examples of these types of drugs include antibiotics, unless taken for prophylactic reasons as prescribed by your physician; pain medications for acute pain, such as after surgery, dental work, or a similar situation; antianxiety medications; antidepressant medications (you may have to take some medications for longer periods of time); seasonal allergy medications; and drugs to treat short-term breathing conditions. You might not need to take these or other medications for more than a few days or weeks, but it depends on you and your symptoms.

The best advice I can give you is to monitor your own symptoms and how you are feeling. If you feel better and are symptom free and can alter other things in your life to avoid taking medications, more power to you! Think about how you felt before you started taking the medication and how you now feel. Is there a difference? Can you be sure that you do not need to take your medication any longer? For example, if you have adult-onset diabetes (type 2) and can lose unwanted pounds, increase your exercising, and alter your diet positively, you may not need to take oral hypoglycemic agents (drugs taken orally to reduce or control blood sugar). Or, if you have high blood pressure and can control your hypertension through diet and exercise and can avoid taking pills, you will be better off.

If you are taking a medication to treat depression (e.g., paroxetine [Paxil], fluoxetine [Prozac], bupropion [Wellbutrin], amitriptyline), do you think that you can continue to feel positively about yourself, be less depressed, and continue without the medication? If your answer is an unequivocal yes, talk to your doctor about perhaps stopping the drug. There is nothing wrong with you if you feel that you still need the medication, but if you can get by without it, it might be something for you to consider.

Do not abruptly stop any of your medications unless you are experiencing a drug interaction. If you do not think you need to continue any of your medications, always check with your pharmacist or physician first.

Think about whether you would be better off without taking your medications. If you can answer yes, ask your doctor about alternatives. If you cannot answer yes, then you may be better off continuing on your medications and trying to be optimally compliant.

Always throw out your expired and old drugs. This may be hard to do because you have paid good money for them. But these outdated drugs can be harmful to you. Have your pharmacist show you on the container how to tell if a drug is still good. Have them tell you which drugs should not be kept, even if you have doses remaining.

Summary

Make it a part of your daily routine to be compliant and take your medications as best you can. Live and thrive by knowing the answers to the questions in this book. If you do not know the answers, find a way to get the answers. Make a determined effort to be compliant, and try to take your drugs as they have been prescribed.

CHAPTER SEVEN

Getting Your Drugs and Drug Taking in Order

Let's Start to Get Our Drug Taking in Order

This chapter will provide you with some information to help you with your drug taking. I want to begin here by covering some things that you should think about with regard to the drugs that you currently take. I would encourage you to seek to limit the number of drugs that you take. Granted, this is not always possible. There may be generic drugs that you can take as well that might save you money. Let me start by going over some things for you to think about when you look at the drugs you take and how you take them.

Take as Few Drugs as Possible

It is always a good practice to take as few drugs as possible. Some physicians who specialize in treating seniors, called gerontologists, recommend reducing the number of drugs you take as much as possible. Some suggest that, when a person is taking eight drugs total per day, before another drug can be added to those prescribed, one drug needs to be stopped. Now this is just a rule of thumb. You may need to take more than eight drugs for very good reasons. This is something that you and your doctor need to discuss and come to agreement on. You should always feel free to ask your doctor to clarify something or to consider something that you suggest. The more you can participate in the decisions concerning your health, the better your health will be and the better the chances are that your drugs will work better too.

Routine Check-Ups

You tune your car and your appliances. You also can fine tune your medicine-taking habits. In other words, have your medicines checked regularly by your doctors and pharmacists. Once every 6 to 12 months, have your doctors and pharmacists review all the drugs that you take. Your pharmacist will know the drugs that you take that come from the pharmacy where they practice but not from elsewhere. So, it is vital that you let your caregivers know what other prescription drugs you are taking from all sources. Your doctors will know what drugs are prescribed by them but not by other doctors or dentists that you see for care. Also, let all your caregivers know the over-the-counter (OTC) drugs you take. These are the drugs that you can buy without a prescription. You may also be taking herbal remedies, vitamin supplements, or tonics; always let your pharmacists and doctors know that you are taking these too. Consumer Reports *OnHealth* suggests that you double-check for needless drugs if you take five or more drugs, have more than three health problems, have several doctors write prescriptions for you, have not reviewed all your drugs and supplements taken with your primary care doctor in the past 6 months, have been hospitalized recently, and/or take a drug for a month or more that can lead to addiction. Addictive drugs might include narcotic pain relievers, drugs to help you sleep at night, or cough syrups that contain codeine or related compounds. Again, your pharmacist can help you with these items too.

Remember What You Read in This Book about Patient Compliance

Patient compliance with medications and regimens is a part of the process of drug use by patients. The prescribed drugs that patients take can be a small part of total drug use by patients. Other drugs taken may include OTC drugs, herbal supplements, vitamins, nutritional supplements, and perhaps drugs borrowed from friends, family members, or strangers. Taking drugs on a regularly scheduled basis is a difficult task. As a matter of fact, 50% of us are not compliant at any one point in time with the drugs that we take. Many things occur in our lives that divert our attention readily to other pressing matters. It is so easy to be critical of ourselves or others who have trouble with taking medications as scheduled. But be easy on yourself! Many times, the dosing and frequency of administration of drugs can be confusing and bewildering.

Various Forms of Patient Compliance

Recall that there are several forms of medication compliance behavior. These range from obtaining your medications after your doctor writes your prescriptions (initial compliance) to taking your drugs as prescribed. The average rate of compliance is 50% across all medication types! You can also be completely compliant and take all of your medications as you should all of the time. Also, you can take too much of your medicines and be hypercompliant (too much of a good thing!).

THE IMPORTANCE OF PATIENT COMPLIANCE BEING THE BEST IT CAN BE

How well you take your medications as prescribed can affect much of your health. The more compliant you are with the drugs that you take, the better your health will be. You may think that you already take too many drugs. However, if you do not take your drugs as prescribed, you will have more health problems and may be prescribed even more drugs. This is why you should take the drugs prescribed for you in the best manner possible. If you take fewer drugs, you will also save money by postponing the need to take other drugs. The more drugs that you take, the more money you will spend. So controlling the drugs that you are taking now allows you to benefit by having better health, lowering costs for drugs, and avoiding other costs in the future. How you take your drugs is called patient compliance with medications and regimens. The prescribed drugs that you take can be a small part of your total drug use. Other drugs taken may include over-the-counter (OTC) drugs, herbal supplements, vitamins, nutritional supplements, and perhaps drugs borrowed from friends, family members, or strangers. For the most part and for most patients, the fewer drugs that you take, the better off you are. This does not mean taking less of the drugs prescribed for you. It means eliminating unnecessary future expenses for more drugs by taking your current drugs in the best manner that you can.

DIFFICULTIES SENIORS FACE WITH MEDICATION COMPLIANCE

Sometimes, it is difficult for seniors to be compliant with the drugs that they take. There are several reasons for this, which are discussed in the following paragraphs.

Social Isolation

Many seniors live alone, and it is hard when you are by yourself to remember when to take your medications. If you happen to live alone, think of a friend who can help you remember to take your drugs. Your friend might be able to call you to remind you to take your medication, and you can do the same for your friend. Work with a "buddy" to help you remember. If you have a relative who lives close to you or who can call you, ask him or her to help you too.

Chronic Disease

As we get older, there are more diseases that we have the potential to get. It is a blessing to have drugs that can prevent complications of disease if we take our medicines correctly. It can make you feel depressed when you have several conditions at the same time (for example, diabetes, high blood pressure, glaucoma, heart failure, etc.). I encourage you to be as well as you can be, even if you have numerous ailments. Taking your drugs as they have been prescribed is a good way to live your best in the health state you are in.

Severity of Disease

When we have chronic diseases for a long period of time, the disease can become more severe over time. This is something that does not need to happen. There are things we can do to limit the outcomes of diseases that become worse and worse. Again, being as compliant as you possibly can be often will help you avoid complications of diseases down the road.

Multiple Drug Regimens

The more ailments we have, often the more drugs are prescribed as a way to treat the diseases. Taking more drugs can lead you to be less compliant than you could be. Again, make it a part of your routine activities to take your drugs at the same time daily.

Complex Drug Regimens

Finally, work with your pharmacist and doctors to help simplify how you take your drugs. It may mean that you can be more compliant by combining the drugs that you take into segments that you can more easily remember. No one can be expected to be compliant 100% of the time. If you slip up and forget a dose, work harder to remember to take your drugs better the next day. Always ask for help, and let others help you try to simplify your drug taking.

Advice on Medication Taking

Always discard your old or unused medications that have expired. Make it a part of your daily routine to take medications at times that will be easy for you to remember. As a result, you will make a habit of taking your drugs at the same time. This might be in the morning, in the evening, or along with another daily task, such as brushing your teeth. It might be in the morning around the time that you eat your breakfast, or it might be at night before you retire in the evening. If it is possible, write down somewhere that you have taken your drugs. This might be on a calendar, in a diary, or in a notebook.

Answers to Know About Your Medications

You should always know several important things about the medications that you take. You can ask your pharmacist for the answer to these questions. Also feel free to ask your doctor to explain the answers to the following questions:

- What is the name of the drug that I am taking?
- What does this drug look like? Are there different forms of this medication?
- What are the generic names for the drugs that I take?
- How should I take the medicine?
- How long should I continue to take the medication?
- What are some side effects that I need to watch out for?
- Will the drugs that I take interact with each other, over-the-counter drugs that I take, or herbal supplements that I take?
- Is there a place that I need to store this medication?
- Does the medication need to be refrigerated?
- Can I take this medication with food, vitamins, or alcoholic beverages?
- What happens if I miss a dose? When should I take the next one?
- When can I expect to see the results of taking this medication?

When dispensed, most prescriptions have as a rule an expiration date that is listed as being 1 year from the date of prescription filling. However, you may be dispensed a drug with a shorter shelf life, and if this is the case, the 1-year date is not correct. You will not know what the original expiration date is unless you ask the pharmacist. Just make sure that the drugs that you are receiving are not expired and correctly marked. Some items, such as ophthalmic (for use in the eyes) or otic (for use in the ears) preparations, have a shorter expiration date due to the way the items are used. As noted, for any ophthalmic preparation, I recommend that after 90 days you discard the remaining amount. You may not have to use the product for this length of time anyway. The tube or ointment may have an extended expiration date listed somewhere on the product itself. However, please note that, once the sterile seal is broken when you open the product for the first time, this expiration date is invalid due to the sterility of the product now being less than listed. The expiration date put on these containers by the manufacturer assumes that the product is unopened and thus remains sterile; once opened, the sterility is lost.

Summary

By getting your drug taking and your drug regimens in order, you can help yourself in a number of ways. You can help postpone additional health problems if you are as compliant as you can be with the number of drugs that you take. If you can help cut down the number of drugs that you take, this will help ease the complexity of the drug regimens that you have. It will also allow you the opportunity to simplify this part of your health care to a better extent.

Anything that we do to improve compliance will rarely be a 100% successful proposition. But most things that we do to become more compliant can improve health for all of us, me included! This should be your goal: to help you and yours become healthier by making the taking of medications easier and thus becoming more compliant with drug regimens. You cannot and should not be expected to do all of this on your own! Your doctors and pharmacists can help you devise the best medicine-taking schedule that you deserve. Ask them to help you, and please be persistent. I have said it before in this book, but you owe it to yourself. And, they owe it to you too!

CHAPTER EIGHT

Over-the-Counter Pain Relief Drugs

Introduction

This chapter will present information about drugs and drug products that you can buy without a prescription that are over-the-counter (OTC) pain medications. Just because a drug can be bought without a prescription does not mean that it is not potentially harmful. The key to any drug, including OTC pain drugs, is to make sure that you can take it and take it safely for the time you should.

Always Check with Your Doctor

Please discuss any and all treatment options with your healthcare professional. The material presented here is for information purposes only; always check with your doctor for specific questions about your health condition.

Over-the-Counter Drugs

As previously noted, OTC drugs are medicines that you can purchase without a prescription in the United States. These are products that the U.S. Food and Drug Administration (FDA) considers to be safe for consumers to use on their own. Always check with your doctor and pharmacist before you begin taking any new product, including drugs that are available over the counter.

OTC Pain Relief

There are several types of pain relief drugs available for you to purchase without a prescription from a doctor. These drugs are called analgesics. Just because these drugs can be bought without a prescription does not mean that they are not real medicines—they are! Always let your caregivers (e.g., doctors, nurses, pharmacists) know if you take any of these drugs. Ask your health providers to let you know which of these drugs might be best for you to take if you need to take a medicine for pain.

Types of OTC Pain Relievers

The types of OTC pain relievers include: aspirin, acetaminophen, and nonsteroidal anti-inflammatory drugs (e.g., ibuprofen, naproxen, and ketoprofen). OTC analgesics such as acetaminophen, aspirin, ibuprofen, ketoprofen, and naproxen are widely used products. They are available at many retail outlets. They are also heavily advertised products in print, on the radio, and on television. As was previously noted, there are "hidden ingredients" in many products. Unless you specifically know that an analgesic is contained in a medication, you may not assume by just looking at the package or name of a product that it contains one of these analgesic medications. It is also very common in the United States for a brand name OTC product to change ingredients but not the name! This can be very confusing for consumers, so always try to know what is in the OTC products that you are taking, and be very cautious about OTC analgesic properties.

Aspirin, ibuprofen, and acetaminophen are three of the most common drugs causing adverse drug reactions in the elderly and are among the top 10 drugs used worldwide. Each of these drugs can be a "hidden ingredient" in many OTC products, which might include:

- Pain relievers
- Cough and cold preparations
- Migraine headache combination products

ASPIRIN

The oldest type of pain reliever is in the class called salicylates. The more common name of the drug used most often is aspirin. Aspirin is contained in many products, and you have to look closely or ask if you do not know what a product contains. For example, the following medications all contain aspirin or a form of aspirin:

- Alka-Seltzer
- Alka-Seltzer Plus
- Pepto-Bismol

- Excedrin
- Pamprin Cramp Caplets

Aspirin is the most common so-called "hidden ingredient" in many OTC products. The above list is not exhaustive; it lists just some of the brand name OTC products that contain a form of aspirin.

Aspirin should be taken very carefully. If you take a blood thinner such as warfarin, you should not take aspirin. In addition to being a drug to relieve pain, aspirin has been shown to reduce the risk of a heart attack or stroke. It is also used as a blood thinner. This action slows down the blood-clotting ability of your body. Aspirin is best taken with food. If you take it on an empty stomach, it can cause an upset stomach. Also, aspirin can cause stomach ulcers when taken over time. If drugs usually do not upset your stomach, aspirin may be an option for you to take for pain relief, headaches, joint pain, arthritis, etc. Aspirin is a pain reliever, decreases the swelling and inflammation of arthritis, and reduces fever.

For the vast majority of persons with asthma, taking aspirin has no effect on their asthma, either good or bad. However, for approximately 3-5% of persons with asthma, aspirin can cause asthma to worsen, often in the form of a severe and sudden attack. Aspirin products should not be used if you consume three or more alcoholic drinks per day.

Aspirin is used chronically for cardiovascular and rheumatologic indications, and many people take the drug in this manner. If you do take a cardioprotective dose of aspirin, please check with your doctor before taking any OTC product for pain relief.

Individuals can also be allergic to aspirin and suffer from rashes, swelling, and have trouble breathing. If you have experienced these reactions in the past while taking aspirin, do not take it again. Also, aspirin can aggravate asthma symptoms and should not be taken by people with asthma.

ACETAMINOPHEN

Acetaminophen is a drug that can relieve pain and reduce a fever. Acetaminophen does not have anti-inflammatory properties. It is important to know that acetaminophen can help with the pain of arthritis, but it cannot reduce swelling. Acetaminophen should not be taken if you drink three or more alcoholic beverages a day. The maximum amount of acetaminophen that you should take in any 24-hour period is eight 500-mg tablets. You can obtain relief from pain with a lower dose than this amount, which is the maximum that anyone should take in a day.

There are numerous prescription products that also contain acetaminophen. You should make sure that you are not taking acetaminophen as an OTC product while also taking a prescription medication that contains acetaminophen. Numerous narcotic pain medications also contain doses of acetaminophen. When in doubt, always check with your pharmacist about what is in the products that you take.

Acetaminophen is available in several dosage forms, including:

- Tablets
- Capsules
- Long-acting capsules that release the drug over an extended period of time
- Capsules meant to dissolve quickly and release the drug very quickly
- Liquid
- Drops
  - Do not measure the drops formulation in a regular dosing cup! Only use the dropper supplied with the original container.
- Suppositories

NONSTEROIDAL ANTI-INFLAMMATORY DRUGS

Nonsteroidal anti-inflammatory drugs (NSAIDs) are a group of drugs that were placed on the market in the 1970s as a prescription-only class of drugs. Later in the 1980s, these drugs were placed in the OTC category. This prescription-to-OTC switch is common in the United States. The strength and dose of these drugs is less than the prescription strength versions. They are serious drugs that should be used carefully.

Please note that people who take NSAIDs (other than aspirin) may have a higher risk of heart attack and stroke than those who do not take these drugs.

Ibuprofen

Ibuprofen was the first of the NSAIDs to be on the market as a prescription drug and the first to be reclassified as an OTC drug as well. The drug is available in a 200-mg strength OTC product. Various companies market ibuprofen in a generic form. The dosage form for ibuprofen can be a:

- Coated caplet
- Coated tablet
- Gelatin-coated tablet
- Liquid-filled gelatin capsule
- Liquid suspension

Ibuprofen is a pain reliever and a drug that can reduce inflammation associated with varying types of arthritis. Ibuprofen can also lower a fever. Ibuprofen should be used after you have consulted your doctor or pharmacist. Ibuprofen can interact with other drugs that you take, and the combination can be too powerful and cause side effects. If you have swelling in your feet or hands, ibuprofen can make this edema worse. If you have heart failure (congestive heart failure), you may experience edema and should not take ibuprofen. Ibuprofen should not be taken with aspirin because the potential for stomach upset or damage is great. You should take no more than six 200-mg tablets in any 24-hour period; this is the maximum dose. It is better if you can take a lower dose and fewer tablets. Ibuprofen and related products should not be used if you consume three or more alcoholic drinks per day.

Naproxen Sodium

Naproxen comes in numerous tablet and capsule formulations manufactured by several companies. Naproxen was introduced as a prescription-only analgesic in the 1970s. It was switched to OTC status several years later. Naproxen is a pain reliever and a drug to reduce inflammation. Naproxen can also work to lower a fever. Naproxen can cause the same type of stomach upset as seen with other NSAIDs. You should not take naproxen along with other analgesic medicines. Do not take more than two 220-mg tablets per day. Do not take naproxen if you drink three or more alcoholic drinks per day. Also, if you notice a rash or swelling, have trouble swallowing, or feel fullness in your throat, call your doctor immediately. If you generally consume three or more alcoholic beverages per day, consult your physician for advice on when and how you should take naproxen or any other pain relievers.

Ketoprofen

Ketoprofen comes in numerous tablet and capsule formulations manufactured by several companies. Ketoprofen was introduced as a prescription-only analgesic in the 1980s. It was switched to OTC status several years later. Ketoprofen is a pain reliever and a drug to reduce inflammation. Ketoprofen can also work to lower a fever. Ketoprofen can cause the same type of stomach upset as seen with other NSAIDs. You should not take ketoprofen along with other analgesic medicines.

The dosage form for Ketoprofen can be an immediate release capsule or a sustained release 24-hour capsule.

If you generally consume three or more alcoholic beverages a day, you should consult your physician for advice on when and how you should take Ketoprofen.

Benefits of OTC NSAID Products

There are many benefits to using OTC NSAID products. For example, consumers can self-diagnose and treat intermittent minor aches and pain without the need for a healthcare provider. Serious adverse events are rare. The majority of consumers use these products safely. The benefits of these therapies outweigh the risks associated with their use. The availability of these ingredients in OTC drug products is not an issue. The FDA believes that these products should remain available as OTC drug products.

As previously noted, NSAIDs can provide effective pain relief. The following list provides examples of categories of pain that can be helped by OTC NSAID products.

- Temporary relief pain
  ○ Headache
  ○ Muscular aches
  ○ Minor pain of arthritis
  ○ Toothache
  ○ Backache
  ○ Common cold
  ○ Menstrual cramps
- Fever

STOMACH BLEEDING WITH BOTH ASPIRIN AND NSAIDs

One of the serious side effects seen with the use of aspirin and NSAIDs is the risk of a dangerous occurrence of stomach bleeding. Risk factors for stomach bleeding as a side effect of NSAID use include the following (Wolfe et al, 1999):

- Previous gastrointestinal bleeding episode; an ulcer due to infection with *Helicobacter pylori* (*H. pylori*)
- Other medical history placing you at risk for a stomach bleed:
  ○ Previous ulcer
  ○ Sensitivity to aspirin or other NSAIDs
- A history of use or overuse of alcohol

- Cigarette smoking
  - Any tobacco use (pipes, chewing tobacco, snuff, cigars, etc.)
- Taking various medications at the same time:
  - NSAID
  - Aspirin
  - Anticoagulant (sodium warfarin)
  - Corticosteroid
    - Prednisone
    - Prednisolone
    - Dexamethasone
- Taking doses of OTC pain medications that are larger than the recommended dose that is present on the labeling for the product
- Advanced age

Always Check Labels

Always check labels of products that you take for colds or the flu. Many of these products contain doses of the pain relievers mentioned here plus other active ingredients. Also be aware that analgesics that are either prescription or OTC drugs do not work as well when individuals smoke. Cigarette smoking impedes the ability of these analgesic drugs to work as well as they would otherwise.

OTC Analgesics in the News

The following is a recall announcement that the U.S. Food and Drug Administration sent out in November 2006 concerning acetaminophen (U.S. Food and Drug Administration, 2006).

FDA Informs Public of Nationwide Recall of 500mg Strength Store-Brand Acetaminophen Caplets

The U.S. Food and Drug Administration (FDA) is alerting the public to a voluntary recall being conducted by Perrigo Company (Perrigo) of Allegan, Michigan for 383 lots of acetaminophen 500mg caplets manufactured and distributed under various store-brands as a result of small metal fragments found in a small number of these caplets. Approximately 11 million bottles containing varying quantities of acetaminophen 500mg caplets are affected by this recall. For a list of batches affected, please see www.fda.gov/oc/po/firmrecalls/perrigo/perrigobatchlist.html. Consumers can determine if they are in possession of a recalled product by locating the batch number printed on the container label. A list of stores that carry store-brands potentially affected by this recall is located on FDA's website at www.fda.gov/oc/po/firmrecalls/perrigo/perrigocustlist.html.

To date, there have been no illness or injuries received related to this problem and no consumer complaints have been reported to the FDA or to Perrigo. Based on information currently available, the FDA believes the probability of serious adverse health consequences is remote; however if a consumer were to swallow an affected caplet, it could result in minor stomach discomfort and/or possible cuts to the mouth or throat. Consumers should consult their physician if they suspect they've been harmed by use of this product.

Consumers who believe they are in possession of the affected products should discontinue use immediately and call Perrigo's Consumer Affairs Department, 877-546-0454 for further instructions. Any adverse reactions experienced with the use of this product should be reported to Perrigo at the above number and the FDA's MedWatch Program by phone at 800-FDA-1088, by fax at 800-FDA-0178 or on the MedWatch website at www.fda.gov/medwatch.

FDA is currently investigating the cause of the metal particles found in the acetaminophen 500 mg. caplets. Perrigo originally informed FDA of this problem after discovering through their own regulatory quality control procedures that their tableting equipment was wearing down prematurely. The company is also investigating the cause of the problem. The ongoing investigations have revealed the presence of the metal fragments in caplets of acetaminophen, 500 mg. Perrigo reported to the FDA that 70 million caplets were passed through a metal detector; resulting in the discovery of approximately 200 caplets containing metal fragments ranging in size from "microdots" to portions of wire 8 mm in length.

At this time FDA does not anticipate that this action will cause a shortage of acetaminophen. Currently, only one strength (500 mg caplets) is affected. Consumers may wish to take additional amounts of the lower strengths of acetaminophen tablets or caplets, which are not affected by this recall, to reach the 500 mg dose or access acetaminophen produced by alternate manufacturers. In all instances, FDA advises consumers to follow labeled instructions for maximum daily dosage.

Perrigo is notifying its distributors and retailers of this issue and will inform them of steps it will take to facilitate product replacement.

Another article released by the FDA in December of 2006 concerns label changes for OTC pain relievers (U.S. Food and Drug Administration, 2006).

FDA Proposes Labeling Changes to Over-the-Counter Pain Relievers

The Food and Drug Administration (FDA) today proposed to amend the labeling regulations on over-the-counter (OTC) Internal Analgesic, Antipyretic, and Antirheumatic (IAAA) drug products to include important safety information regarding the potential for stomach bleeding and liver damage and when to consult a doctor. OTC IAAA drug products, commonly known as acetaminophen and nonsteroidal anti-inflammatory drugs (NSAIDs), such as aspirin, ibuprofen, naproxen and ketoprofen, are used to treat pain, fever, headaches, and muscle aches.

To help ensure safe use of OTC products, and to provide consumers with the labeling necessary for them to make more informed medical decisions, FDA is proposing the following label changes:

For Products Containing Acetaminophen

- *To require new warnings which would highlight the potential for liver toxicity, particularly when using acetaminophen in high doses, when taking more than one product with acetaminophen, and when taken with moderate amounts of alcohol;*
- *To require that the ingredient acetaminophen be prominently identified on the product's principal display panel (PDP) of the immediate container, and the outer carton (if applicable).*

For Products Containing NSAIDs

- *To require new warnings for products that contain an NSAID which would highlight the potential for stomach bleeding in persons over age 60, in persons who have had prior ulcers or bleeding, in persons who*

Over-the-Counter Pain Relief Drugs

take a blood thinner, when taking more than one product containing an NSAID, when taken with moderate amounts of alcohol, and when taking for longer time than directed; and

- *To require that the name of the NSAID ingredient and the term "NSAID" be prominently identified on the product's PDP of the immediate container and the outer carton (if applicable).*

The new labeling would be required for all OTC drug products that contain only an IAAA ingredient, as well as for products that contain an IAAA ingredient with other ingredients, such as cold symptom relievers. Consumers may also be taking IAAA ingredients in their prescription medications, which makes it important to alert them of the contents of their OTC medications, so they do not take too much of an IAAA ingredient.

FDA based its proposal for labeling changes on previous Advisory Committee discussions, recommendations, and public comments (see http://www .fda.gov/ohrms/dockets/ac/cder02.htm#NonprescriptionDrugs) and a review of the scientific literature.

A number of manufacturers of OTC internal analgesic drug products already have voluntarily implemented labeling changes to identify these potential safety concerns.

Between now and when these recommendations are implemented, no doubt other OTC makers will do the same thing. Then all these products with these ingredients will have uniform requirements for labeling that should help many people become better informed and hopefully achieve the relief that these products promote.

Individual and Combination Products

Many individual and combination products containing acetaminophen, aspirin, and ibuprofen are available as OTC and/or prescription-only products. I have compiled several listings of the individual and combination products that are available. Please note that these listings are by no means complete because there are many such products available. Please see the following tables:

Table 8-1. Acetaminophen OTC Products. Adapted from Clinical Pharmacology Online, 2007.

Table 8-2. Acetaminophen-Containing Prescription Products. Adapted from Clinical Pharmacology Online, 2007.

Table 8-3. Some of the Products on the Market That Contain Aspirin. Adapted from Clinical Pharmacology Online, 2007.

Table 8-4. Selected Prescription and OTC Combination Products That Contain Aspirin. Adapted from Clinical Pharmacology Online, 2007.

Table 8-5. Ibuprofen-Containing OTC Individual and Combination Products. Adapted from Clinical Pharmacology Online, 2007.

Table 8-6. Ibuprofen-Containing Prescription Products. Adapted from Clinical Pharmacology Online, 2007.

Table 8-1   Acetaminophen OTC Products

Acephen	Genapap Extra Strength	T-Painol Extra Strength
Aceta	Genebs	T-Panol
Actamin	Infantaire	Tempra 1
Adprin B	Liquiprin	Tempra 2
Anacin AF	Lopap	Tempra 3
Anacin-3 Maximum Strength	Mapap	Tycolene
	Mapap Junior Strength	Tylenol
Apacet	Mardol	Tylenol 8 Hour
Apra	Masophen	Tylenol Arthritis
Apra Cherry	Neopap Supprettes	Tylenol Children's
Apra Grape	O-Pap	Tylenol Infants
Children's Pain and Fever	Pain-Eze	Tylenol Junior
Children's Silapap	Panadol	Tylenol Sore Throat
Comtrex Sore Throat Relief	Panadol Jr.	Tylenol Sore Throat Daytime
	Q-Pap	
Dolono	Q-Pap Extra Strength	Tylophen
Dolono Infant	Redutemp	Uni-Ace
Ed-APAP	Ridenol	Uni-Ace Child
ElixSure Fever/Pain	S-T Febrol	Uniserts
Equate Pain Reliever	St. Joseph Aspirin-Free	Vitapap
Feverall	T-Painol	XS No Aspirin PR
Genapap		XS Pain Reliever

Source: Clinical Pharmacology Online, 2007.

Table 8-2   Acetaminophen-Containing Prescription Products

Acetaminophen; butalbital

Acetaminophen; butalbital; caffeine

Acetaminophen; butalbital; caffeine; codeine

Acetaminophen; caffeine; chlorpheniramine; hydrocodone; phenylephrine

Acetaminophen; caffeine; dihydrocodeine

Acetaminophen; caffeine; magnesium salicylate; phenyltoloxamine

Acetaminophen; caffeine; phenyltoloxamine; salicylamide

Acetaminophen; codeine

Acetaminophen; dextromethorphan; doxylamine

Acetaminophen; dextromethorphan; doxylamine; pseudoephedrine

Acetaminophen; dichloralphenazone; isometheptene

Acetaminophen; hydrocodone

Acetaminophen; oxycodone

Acetaminophen; pamabrom

Acetaminophen; pamabrom; pyrilamine

Acetaminophen; pentazocine

Acetaminophen; phenyltoloxamine

Acetaminophen; propoxyphene

Acetaminophen; tramadol

Hydrocodone; acetaminophen

Source: Clinical Pharmacology Online, 2007.

Table 8-3   Some of the Products on the Market That Contain Aspirin

Acuprin 81

Adult Low Strength Enteric Coated Aspirin

Arthritis Pain

Ascriptin Enteric

Aspergum Orginal

Aspir-Low

Aspir-trin

Aspirin

Aspirin Child

Aspirin Child Chewable

Aspirin Enteric Coated

Aspirin Litecoat

Aspirin Lo-Dose

Aspirin Low Strength

Aspirin, ASA

Aspirtab

Bayer

Bayer Children's

Bayer Low Strength

Bayer Migraine Pain

Bayer Plus

Bayer Therapy

Bayer Women's

Child Aspirin

Children's Chewable Aspirin

Easprin

Ecotrin

Ecotrin Maximum Strength

Empirin

Entercote

Enteric Coated Regular Strength Aspirin

Extra Strength Coated Aspirin

Genacote

Gennin FC

Genprin

Halfprin

Litecoat Aspirin

Low Dose Adult Aspirin

Minitabs

Norwich Aspirin

Ridiprin

Safety Coated Aspirin 81 mg

St. Joseph Aspirin

St. Joseph Aspirin Adult Chewable

St. Joseph Aspirin Adult EC

Stanback Analgesic

Uni-Tren

Zero Order Aspirin

ZORprin

Source: Clinical Pharmacology Online, 2007.

Table 8-4   Selected Prescription and OTC Combination Products That Contain Aspirin

Aspirin, ASA; butalbital; caffeine	Aspirin, ASA; carisoprodol; codeine
Aspirin, ASA; butalbital; caffeine; codeine	Aspirin, ASA; codeine
Aspirin, ASA; caffeine	Aspirin, ASA; diphenhydramine
Aspirin, ASA; caffeine; dihydrocodeine	Aspirin, ASA; dipyridamole
Aspirin, ASA; caffeine; orphenadrine	Aspirin, ASA; hydrocodone
Aspirin, ASA; caffeine; propoxyphene	Aspirin, ASA; meprobamate
Aspirin, ASA; caffeine; salicylamide	Aspirin, ASA; methocarbamol
Aspirin, ASA; calcium carbonate; magnesium oxide; magnesium carbonate	Aspirin, ASA; oxycodone
	Aspirin, ASA; pentazocine
Aspirin, ASA; carisoprodol	Aspirin, ASA; pravastatin

Source: Clinical Pharmacology Online, 2007.

Table 8-5   Ibuprofen-Containing OTC Individual and Combination Products

Children's Ibuprofen	Ibuprofen Children's
Chlorpheniramine; ibuprofen; pseudoephedrine	Ibuprofen Cold and Sinus
Diphenhydramine; ibuprofen	Ibuprofen IB
Equate Children's Ibuprofen Cold	Ibuprofen Junior Strength
Equate Ibuprofen Cold and Sinus	Ibuprofen lysine
Ibuprofen	Ibuprofen, Jr.
	Ibuprofen; pseudoephedrine

Source: Clinical Pharmacology Online, 2007.

Table 8-6   Ibuprofen-Containing Prescription Products

Hydrocodone; ibuprofen
Ibuprofen 600 mg or greater dose per unit
Ibuprofen; oxycodone

Source: Clinical Pharmacology Online, 2007.

Summary

OTC analgesic products are widely available for consumers to buy and use. They are safe for consumers to take provided the labeled directions are followed and the recommended dose is not exceeded. Some individuals should not take these products because of prior adverse effects or a previous stomach bleeding occurrence. Your doctor can help you decide which, if any, of these products might be best for you. Many of these analgesic products are also ingredients in other OTC products for cold and flu symptoms, and they have many different names. I mentioned this hidden ingredient aspect of these products earlier. Always know what the ingredients are in the medicines that you take. If you have a question about ingredients, always know that you can ask your pharmacist a question about these products at any time in any pharmacy.

References

U.S. Food and Drug Administration. FDA informs public of nationwide recall of 500mg strength store-brand acetaminophen caplets. November 9, 2006. Available at http://www.fda.gov/bbs/topics/NEWS/2006/NEW01507.html; accessed March 16, 2006.

U.S. Food and Drug Administration. FDA proposes labeling changes to over-the-counter pain relievers. December 19, 2006. Available at http://www.fda.gov/bbs/topics/NEWS/2006/NEW01533.html; accessed March 16, 2006.

Wolfe MM, Lichtenstein DR, Singh G. Gastrointestinal toxicity of nonsteroidal antiinflammatory drugs. *N Engl J Med.* 1999;340:1888–1899.

CHAPTER NINE

Drug–Drug Interactions

Introduction

This chapter will present information about interactions that can occur between the drugs that you take for your health conditions. When one drug is taken with another drug and alters the actions of the drug, a drug interaction is said to occur. Any drug can interact with another drug and cause problems that range from minor to severe. The interaction depends on the drug and what it is taken with. The activity of a drug can be affected by foods, beverages, over-the-counter (OTC) medications, or other prescription medications.

Always Check with Your Doctor

Please discuss any and all treatment options with your healthcare professional. The material presented here is for information purposes only; always check with your doctor for specific questions about your health condition.

Why Drug Interactions Are Important

Impact of Aging and Different Disease States

As we grow older, it is very common to have several different disease states. These may include:

- Hypertension
- Congestive heart failure
- Diabetes mellitus
- Arthritis
- Depression
- Osteoporosis
- Acid-peptic disease

Drug–Drug Interactions

The Use of Drugs

A common way to treat these conditions is with prescription medications. When several prescription medications are taken at the same time, drug interactions may possibly occur. Several things can happen when two or more drugs are taken together; some possibilities are as follows:

- Sometimes when drugs are taken together, they can work like they always work; that is, there is no negative consequence from taking the drugs together.
- In some cases, when two or more drugs are taken together, one or both drugs may have an exaggerated effect; that is, they work together too well. This type of interaction is called a synergistic reaction.
- In other cases, when two drugs are taken at the same time, the drugs may counteract one another and will not work as they normally would work alone.

How to Prepare for Taking Drugs

There are things that you can do to prepare for how you will respond to the drugs that you take. These action include the following:

- Always consult your doctor and pharmacist before you take any drug.
- Learn about the purpose and actions of all drugs prescribed.
- Learn about the possible side effects of the drugs.
- Learn how to take your drugs and how to deal with the possible side effects of the drugs.
- Report to the doctor or pharmacist any symptoms that might be related to the use of a drug.
- If you are seeing more than one doctor, make sure each doctor knows all the drugs being taken.

Occurrence of Drug Interactions

Drug interactions can occur with any and all medications or herbs that are consumed. As a general rule, drugs from the same class of drugs should not be taken together, and drugs that are used to treat the same ailment should not generally be taken at the same time. This is true regardless of whether the drug is an antibiotic, a drug to treat arthritis (such as nonsteroidal anti-inflammatory drugs [NSAIDs] or cyclo-oxygenase-2 [COX-2] inhibitors), an oral hypoglycemic drug, a diuretic, a drug to treat depression, a drug to treat anxiety, or a drug to help you sleep. Pain medications should also not be combined. Pain medications and drugs to treat anxiety or depression should be used together cautiously, if used together at all. The effects of these combined drugs are just too intense, and it is not safe to combine them. Never take drugs from the same class together, whether they are prescription or OTC products or both prescription and OTC products.

Some drugs may be prescribed by your doctor in combination because they may make each other work better (synergism) in a positive fashion. An example might be drugs to treat pain (narcotic analgesics or others) and a tricyclic antidepressant (TCA) such as amitriptyline (Elavil), or an antidepressant such as doxepin (Sinequan). Please do not combine these drugs unless your doctor has ordered them both for you.

Types of Interactions

Pseudoephedrine and Phenylephrine

Drugs such as pseudoephedrine (Sudafed) or phenylephrine (Sudafed PE) can interact with drugs called monoamine oxidase (MAO) inhibitors, leading to an excessive high blood pressure (malignant hypertension). These drugs should never be taken in combination (Fincham, 2005). Ask your pharmacist or physician for more guidance. MAO inhibitors include the following:

- Isocarboxazid (Marplan)
- Phenelzine (Nardil)
- Tranylcyopromine (Parnate)

The combination of pseudoephedrine or phenylephrine with MAO inhibitors can lead to severe headache, high blood pressure, high fever, and/or hypertensive crisis (life-threatening increase in blood pressure).

Thyroid Hormones

Thyroid hormones such as levothyroxine (Synthroid), liothyronine (e.g., Cytomel), liotrix (Thyrolar), and thyroid (e.g., Armour Thyroid) should not be taken with anticoagulants (sodium warfarin or anisindione) (Lacy et al, 2004). The anticoagulant effect of warfarin may be increased, causing bleeding episodes, if taken with thyroid hormones. A solution to this interaction could be to have your doctor decrease the dose of the anticoagulant that you are taking. This is a decision your doctor will need to make.

Methotrexate

Drugs that are taken for arthritis often upset your stomach. Taking these drugs plus a cancer drug like methotrexate can cause serious stomach upset, ulcers, or bleeding. See Table 9-1 for a list of drugs that should not be used with methotrexate (Lacy et al, 2004).

Anticoagulants

Drugs called anticoagulants (sodium warfarin [Coumadin]) should not be taken with the antibiotics listed below (Anonymous, 2004):

- Azithromycin
- Clarithromycin

Table 9-1   Nonsteroidal Anti-Inflammatory Drugs That Can Interact with Methotrexate

Diclofenac	Ketoprofen	Naproxen
Etodolac	Ketorolac	Oxaprozin
Fenoprofen	Meclofenamate	Piroxicam
Ibuprofen	Mefanamic acid	Sulindac
Indomethacin	Nabumetone	Tolmetin

- Dirithromycin
- Erythromycin
- Troleandomycin
- Fluoroquinolones

Statin Drugs

The class of drugs called statins, which are used to treat high cholesterol or lipid levels, should not be taken with:

- Nefazodone
- Macrolide antibiotics
- Sodium warfarin and anticoagulants

Alcohol

Consumption of alcoholic beverages by persons with diabetes can make control of the person's blood sugar difficult. Insulin does not work as well when persons with diabetes drink alcoholic beverages. There is an enhanced level of activity of the insulin when used along with alcoholic beverages. This makes the sugar-lowering effect of diabetes more pronounced (hypoglycemia, or low blood sugar). If alcohol is consumed, it might be best to always check with your physician. Drinking alcohol in smaller amounts or with a meal or snack might be an option that your physician might approve.

Other Reactions

Other effects can also be severe; examples of these interactions are prevalent and include synergistic reactions occurring between prescription and OTC medications. The following is an example of an effect that is synergistic. A patient may be stabilized on the drug warfarin (Coumadin), which is taken for blood clots or clotting disorders. This patient may then self-medicate with OTC aspirin. The effect of the aspirin plus warfarin is greater than the effect of either drug taken alone, and thus, the patient may have excess bleeding due to the synergistic effect of the combination of these two drugs. Unless the patient has specifically been counseled by either the physician or pharmacist to not take the warfarin with aspirin, the patient may inadvertently run into bleeding troubles by consuming both at the same time.

Laxatives

Sometimes two seemingly simple medications should not be taken at the same time because severe and serious interactions could possibly occur. There are two commonly used laxatives—docusate and mineral oil. The two laxatives interact severely and negatively. Docusate is a stool softener and mild laxative. Mineral oil is a stronger laxative that has more of a purgative effect. Mineral oil can also be included in other laxatives, so it may be a hidden ingredient (again, you really need to know what is in the products you take). When these two laxatives are taken together, the mineral oil may be absorbed into the bloodstream, whereas when taken alone, the mineral oil cannot be absorbed into the bloodstream. The docusate (DSS) transforms the mineral oil into small particles that can be absorbed. These small emulsified globules can then enter the lungs from the bloodstream and lead to a very serious form of pneumonia called lipoid pneumonia. Therefore, be cautious about combining drugs without asking your pharmacist first. Because these and similar products are obtained without a prescription (e.g., they are OTCs), your pharmacist may not know what you are taking unless you ask beforehand and inform the pharmacist of all the drugs you are taking.

There are some laxatives that are not meant to dissolve in the upper gastrointestinal (GI) tract (the stomach) but, instead, are meant to dissolve in the intestines. The stomach itself has an acidic pH (allows foods to dissolve), whereas the lower GI tract has a basic pH. The pH level determines whether a substance is termed acidic or basic. Drugs can be formulated so that they dissolve in the lower GI tract alone. These drugs, called enteric-coated, bypass the acidic environment of the upper GI tract and can dissolve easily in the lower GI tract. If some drugs are caustic and capable of producing stomach upset, they are coated in such a fashion as to dissolve in the intestines. Bisacodyl tablets (Dulcolax) are an example of an enteric-coated product. Bisacodyl oral tablets should not be taken with items that will make the upper stomach have a more basic pH level. Thus, bisacodyl tablets should not be taken with milk or milk products or with antacid preparations. These tablets should also never be cut in half in order to save money. Again, the medication itself is caustic to the walls of the upper GI tract.

Use Your Pharmacist!

Always check with your pharmacist to see whether several drugs can be taken at the same time. Before you take a drug for congestion that is called a nasal decongestant (Sudafed) to help with a cold or nasal stuffiness, ask your doctor or pharmacist about using the product if you have any of the following conditions:

- Diabetes
- Hypertension
- Cardiac disease
- Prostate disease
- Thyroid disease

Drugs for Erectile Dysfunction (Male Impotence)

Drugs for erectile dysfunction (phosphodiesterase inhibitors [Viagra, Cialis, Levitra]) SHOULD NOT be taken with the following drugs for heart conditions:

- Amyl nitrate
- Isosorbide dinitrate
- Isosorbide mononitrate
- Nitroglycerin sublingual tablets, patch, or ointment

Metronidazole

Metronidazole (Flagyl) is an antiprotozoal anti-infective drug. It is available by prescription only and often used to treat the infection caused by the parasite Trichomonas. Metronidazole *should never* be taken with alcohol. The combination produces what is termed a disulfiram-type reaction. Disulfiram (Antabuse) is a drug used to help alcoholics avoid relapse. Alcohol in combination with disulfiram causes violent stomach upset, severe flushing, fever, chills, severe shaking, and general discomfort. Patients who participate in disulfiram therapy *knowingly* take the drug recognizing that it is a self-administered deterrent to going back to drinking, and they know that if they do drink and take the drug, they will have a certain and negative reaction immediately.

Know What Your Drugs Do and How They Work

The more you know about drugs, the safer you are. The following are some of the most commonly prescribed medications and their interactions with other substances:

- Antidiarrheals (atropine and diphenoxylate [Lomotil]): Used to treat diarrhea, Lomotil can increase the effect of tranquilizers, sleeping pills, and sedatives. Loperamide (Imodium A-D) can have the same affect on these central nervous system (CNS) depressants.
- Antihistamines: The sedative effect of the older antihistamines (even OTC varieties such as diphenhydramine and chlorpheniramine) can be increased by drinking alcoholic beverages or taking other medicines containing alcohol.
- Aspirin: Taken for its pain-relieving and blood-thinning properties, aspirin taken with alcohol can cause the stomach lining to bleed.
- Penicillin/ampicillin: The effectiveness of these drugs, which are used to treat infections, can be reduced when they are taken with food. Take these antibiotics 1 hour before meals or 2 hours after meals.

- Sleeping pills: Many seniors find that they have difficulty sleeping as they get older and take OTC or prescription sleeping pills. However, if taken with alcohol, sleeping pills can cause extreme drowsiness, coma, and even death.
- Tranquilizers: Some aging authorities believe that the elderly take far too many tranquilizers for everything from depression to chronic pain. Like sleeping pills, when tranquilizers are taken with alcohol, they can cause drowsiness, unconsciousness, coma, and death.

Alcohol and Drugs

Individuals who consume three or more alcoholic beverages should not take OTC or prescription medications that contain acetaminophen, aspirin, or ibuprofen (or other nonsteroidal anti-inflammatory drugs).

Effects of Cigarette Smoking on Drugs

Cigarettes have a negative effect on virtually all medications. Drugs simply do not work as well when someone smokes.

There are many identified interactions between smoking and medications. One type of interaction, the effect of smoking on drug metabolism, is well documented. The primary mechanism for interactions appears to be the induction of liver enzymes by compounds present in tobacco smoke. Smokers should use caution when taking the following drugs:

- Clozapine (Clozaril) is a drug to treat schizophrenia, and when used by a smoker, a higher dose may need to be administered.
- Beta-blockers (β-blockers) do not work as well in treating patients with blood pressure or cardiac arrhythmias who smoke.
- Insulin is not as well absorbed in smokers, and it may be necessary to increase the amount of insulin used.

- When used by a smoker, warfarin is cleared from the system quicker, plasma concentrations are decreased, and thus higher doses may be necessary.
- Smokers who take tricyclic antidepressants (e.g., amitriptyline [Elavil, Endep], nortriptyline [Pamelor, Aventil], imipramine [Tofranil]) have lower levels of the drugs, and the drugs may not work as well.
- Female smokers who continue to smoke while taking female hormones (estrogen) run the risk of heart attack, stroke, and deep vein thrombosis.
  - Estrogen is the interacting drug, and thus, postmenopausal women who take estrogen supplementation and continue to smoke run the risk as well. Smokers should not use estrogen products.
- As noted in the previous chapter, pain medications, either prescription or OTC, do not work as well when individuals smoke.

Alternate therapy may be available for some patients who cannot stop smoking. For example, the ulcer patient could instead take sucralfate. It does not influence acid production but rather coats the site of ulceration with a spongy film, thus allowing the ulcerated lesion to heal. However, if the patient continues to smoke, healing will be delayed. Patients who have other conditions and who stop smoking may need to decrease their medication dosages (e.g., diabetes patients who take insulin or patients who take theophylline).

Summary

The precise mechanisms of the interactions mentioned in this chapter remain unclear. It is not known whether the effect is caused by tobacco substrates (nicotine or others) or by other byproducts of smoking (polycyclic aromatic hydrocarbons). Nevertheless, it is important for patients to be aware of what is occurring and why. They may try to stop smoking if they can be convinced that it is futile to try to influence other disease states and attendant drug therapies while continuing

Drug–Drug Interactions

to smoke. Despite a medication's demonstrated efficacy in nonsmokers or appropriate compliance by the smoking patient, the negative health effects of smoking and the associated lack of response to the medication can eventually overcome and negate any drug therapy.

When drugs enhance the action of another drug, the effects of the combination may be much more intense than either effect alone. For instance, when diphenhydramine (Benadryl), an antihistamine, and a sleep medication such as triazolam (Halcion) are taken at the same time, increased drowsiness can occur. Each can cause drowsiness alone (the triazolam is taken to induce sleep), but the combination can make a person even more drowsy (sleepy). I would not recommend that these two drugs be taken together. There are nonsedating antihistamines that do not cause drowsiness for most folks. These nonsedating antihistamines include loratadine (Claritin), desloratadine (Clarinex), cetirizine (Zyrtec), acrivastine and pseudoephedrine hydrochloride (Semprex), and fexofenadine (Allegra).

As noted, taking a sedating antihistamine with alcohol will intensify the effect of each of the two substances. The same is true for alcohol taken with a drug to reduce anxiety such as diazepam, lorazepam, or another similar drug.

It is important to recognize that any drug can interact with other drugs. Patients need to ask pharmacists questions and tell caregivers all the drugs they take.

References

Anonymous. Drug interaction reminder—fluoroquinolone antibiotics and the anticoagulant (blood thinner) warfarin (Coumadin). *Worst Pills Best Pills* 2004;10: 70-71.

Fincham JE. Taking Your Medicine: A Guide to Medication Regimens and Compliance for Patients and Caregivers. New York: Pharmaceutical Products Press, Inc., 2005, pp 69-70.

Lacy CF, et al. Lexi-Comp's Drug Information Handbook 2004-2005. 12th ed. Hudson, OH: Lexi-Comp Inc., 2004, pp 945, 1521.

CHAPTER TEN

Drug–Herbal Product Interactions

Introduction

In this chapter, I will present information about interactions that can occur between the drugs that you take for your health conditions and herbal supplements that you might also be taking. When one drug is taken with another drug and this alters the actions of the drugs, a drug interaction is said to occur. Any drug can interact with another drug and cause problems that range from minor to severe. The interaction depends on the drugs and what they are taken with. The activity of a drug can be affected by foods, beverages, over-the-counter (OTC) medications, vitamins and minerals, herbal products, or other prescription medications.

Always Check with Your Doctor

Please discuss any and all treatment options with your healthcare professional. The material presented here is for information purposes only; always check with your doctor for specific questions about your health condition.

Drug Interactions

When several prescription medications are taken at the same time, drug interactions may possibly occur. Several things can happen when two or more drugs are taken together; some possibilities are as follows:

- Sometimes when drugs are taken together, they can work like they always work; that is, there is no negative consequence from taking the drugs together.
- In some cases, when two or more drugs are taken together, one or both drugs may have an exaggerated effect; that is, they work together too well. This type of interaction is called a synergistic reaction.

- In other cases, when two drugs are taken at the same time, the drugs may counteract one another and will not work as they normally would work alone.

What Can You Do to Get the Most from Your Therapies?

There are things you can do to help prepare for how you will respond to the drugs and herbal supplements that you take. These items include:

- Always consult your doctor and pharmacist before you take any drug.
- Learn about the purpose and actions of all drugs prescribed.
- Learn about the possible side effects of the drugs.
- Learn how to take your drugs and how to deal with the possible side effects of the drugs
- Report to the doctor or pharmacist any symptoms that might be related to the use of a drug.
- If you are seeing more than one doctor, make sure each doctor knows all of the drugs you are taking.

Also please always remember that:

- Any drug can interact with other drugs.
- Patients need to check with pharmacists for questions.
- Patients need to tell caregivers all of the drugs they take.
- Drug interactions can occur with any and all medications, herbs, or drugs that are consumed.

Types of Drugs

Let me just briefly outline the different drug types and give some examples from each class of drugs (please note, the lists of drug examples do not contain all of the drugs available within the classes of drugs):

Prescription Drugs

- Prescription drugs
  - These are the medicines that your doctor prescribes for you that require you to have a prescription; some examples of conditions for which prescription drugs would be prescribed include the following:
  −High blood pressure
  −Diabetes
  −Antibiotics
  −Cancer drugs
  −Osteoporosis
  −Arthritis

Over-the-Counter Drugs

- Over-the-counter (OTC) drugs
  - Acetaminophen (Tylenol and countless other generic and brand name products)
  - Aspirin (Bayer and countless other generic and brand name products)

Herbal Supplements

- Herbal supplements
  - Alfalfa
  - Echinacea
  - Feverfew
  - Garlic (for medicinal and not kitchen applications)
  - Ginkgo balboa
  - Ginseng
  - Kava-kava
  - Lemon balm
  - Licorice
  - St. John's wort
  - Valerian
  - Many, many others

Social Drugs

- Social drugs (please note that all of these substances can interact with the other medications that you might be taking)
  - Caffeine
  - Alcohol
  - Nicotine, from cigarettes, pipes, cigars, chewing tobacco, etc.

Specific Interactions

I would like to briefly discuss some specific interactions that have occurred between herbal supplements and other drugs that you might be taking.

St. John's Wort

The flowering tops of St. John's wort are used to prepare teas and tablets containing concentrated extracts. St. John's wort is a commonly used herbal product that has an adverse effect on many drugs. It is used by many individuals without their physicians' knowledge to treat depression, but St. John's wort *has not* been proven to be effective at treating depression (Drug interactions with St. John's wort, 2000). The supplement has been shown to decrease the effectiveness of warfarin (increased potential for bleeding episodes) and to result in lower blood levels of amitriptyline (an antidepressant) and lower blood levels of the heart failure drug digoxin. St. John's wort may cause increased sensitivity to sunlight. In addition, a photosensitivity reaction (severe reaction to sun or light exposure) has been shown (The University of Michigan Health System, 2007) when St. John's wort was taken with piroxicam (Feldene), a prescription NSAID. Other side effects can include anxiety, dry mouth, dizziness, gastrointestinal symptoms, fatigue, headache, and sexual dysfunction.

St. John's wort has also been shown to lower blood levels of simvastatin (a cholesterol-lowering drug) and cyclosporine (a drug taken to reduce the potential for rejection with organ transplantations)

(Fincham, 2005). It has also been shown to cause grogginess when taken with the antidepressant drug paroxetine (Prozac) and to lead to serotonin syndrome when taken with other selective serotonin reuptake inhibitors (SSRIs) or with pseudoephedrine (Sudafed) (Fincham). Lower blood levels of the antiasthmatic drug theophylline have occurred when taken with St. John's wort (Fincham). The blood levels of the drug class benzodiazepines have also been shown to be decreased when taking St. John's wort at the same time (Fincham). Thus, St. John's wort has the potential to lessen the effectiveness for these drugs. Benzodiazepines include:

- Alprazolam (Xanax)
- Clonazepam (Klonapin)
- Diazepam (Valium)
- Midazolam (Versed)
- Triazolam (Halcion)

Anyone who may have depression should see a healthcare provider. There are effective proven therapies available. It is important to inform your healthcare providers about any herb or dietary supplement you are using, including St. John's wort. This helps to ensure safe and coordinated care.

Echinacea (*Echinacea augustifolia*)

Echinacea is an herb promoted to treat the symptoms of a cold or flu. Echinacea should not be taken with ketoconazole (Nizoral) or methotrexate since the combination can lead to liver toxicity (Fincham, 2005). Echinacea should also not be taken with immunosuppressant drugs such as:

- Azathioprine (Imuran)
- Cyclosporine (Neoral, Sandimmune)
- Tacrolimus (Prograf)

If echinacea is taken with immunosuppressant drugs, it may reduce their effectiveness (Fincham, 2005).

Alfalfa (*Medicago sativa*)

Alfalfa may be taken to treat symptoms of arthritis, asthma, stomach upset, or high cholesterol. Alfalfa should not be taken with anticoagulants (sodium warfarin). Alfalfa contains coumarin components and thus may make the activity of warfarin stronger (Fincham, 2005).

Feverfew (*Tanacetum parthenium*)

Feverfew is an herb promoted to treat migraine headaches, fever, or perhaps menstrual difficulties. Feverfew should not be taken with anticoagulants (sodium warfarin) because it may enhance the effect of warfarin and lead to enhanced bleeding (Fincham, 2005).

Garlic (*Allium sativum*)

Garlic as an herbal product (not a spice or cooking aid) has been promoted to treat high cholesterol, high blood pressure, and other cardiac ailments. Garlic should not be taken with anticoagulants (sodium warfarin) due to the potentiation of the effect of warfarin; this may lead to bleeding episodes (Fincham, 2005).

Ginkgo (*Ginkgo biloba*)

Ginkgo is an herbal product variously suggested to help symptoms of varicose veins, intermittent claudication (leg pains due to poor circulation), vertigo (dizziness), tinnitus (ringing in the ears), or SSRI-induced sexual dysfunction. Ginkgo should not be taken with anticoagulants (sodium warfarin) because this may lead to bleeding episodes (Fincham, 2005). Ginkgo should also not be taken with anticonvulsants (e.g., phenytoin, carbamazepine); this combination may lead to less effectiveness of the seizure medications and thus cause an increase in seizures (Fincham, 2005).

Ginseng (*Panax quinquefolium*)

Ginseng is an herbal supplement promoted to reduce stress. Ginseng should not be used with anticoagulants (sodium warfarin); this may lead to bleeding episodes (Fincham, 2005). Ginseng should not be taken with oral hypoglycemic drugs (see Chapter 9) because it may enhance the effects of the oral diabetes medications as ginseng has a potentially similar effect (Fincham). Ginseng should not be taken with furosemide because it may reduce the effectiveness of the diuretic (Fincham). Ginseng should not be taken with digoxin because it may lower the blood levels of digoxin (Fincham). Ginseng should also not be taken with monoamine oxidase (MAO) inhibitors (see Chapter 9) because it may increase psychoactive stimulation (hallucinations) (Fincham).

Kava-Kava (*Piper methysticum*)

Kava-kava is an herbal supplement promoted to treat anxiety or sleep disorders. This supplement should not be taken with other drugs that also may cause drowsiness or have a sedative effect because these drugs, such as alcoholic beverages or benzodiazepines (see Chapter 9), which are used to treat anxiety or to help in sleep disorders (insomnia), may have a more pronounced effect when taken with kava-kava (Fincham, 2005).

Lemon Balm (*Melissa officinalis L.*)

Lemon balm is an herbal supplement that has been promoted to treat insomnia and anxiety. This herb should not be taken with other drugs that cause central nervous system depression (e.g., antianxiety agents, alcohol, etc.) because it can have an additive effect with these drugs (Fincham, 2005). Lemon balm should also not be taken with thyroid hormones (see Chapter 9) because it can lessen the effectiveness of the thyroid therapy (Fincham, 2005).

Licorice (*Glycyrrhiza glabra*)

Licorice has been suggested to help ulcers and help as an expectorant (removing phlegm). Licorice is also a popular candy. In *any* form, licorice should not be taken with spironolactone (Aldactone, Aldactazide), a diuretic (Fincham, 2005). Licorice actually antagonizes the effect of the diuretic. Licorice should also not be taken with digoxin (Fincham) because it may cause low potassium levels (hypokalemia), thus affecting the cardiac effects of digoxin (Fincham). Licorice should also not be taken with MAO inhibitors (See Chapter 9) because licorice contains drug products called sympathomimetic amines, and the combination may lead to a serious condition termed hypertensive crisis, which is an abnormally high level of blood pressure (Fincham).

Valerian (*Valeriana officinalis*)

Valerian is promoted for use to treat anxiety. When valerian is taken with other central nervous system depressants (e.g., alcohol, opiate pain medications, barbiturates, or other depressants), there can be a sedative additive effect (Fincham, 2005). Barbiturates include the following:

- Amobarbital (Amytal)
- Aprobarbital (Alurate)
- Butabarbital (Butisol)
- Butalbital
- Mephobarbital (Mebaral)
- Pentobarbital (Nembutal)
- Phenobarbital
- Primidone (Mysoline)
- Secobarbital (Seconal)

How to Reduce the Risk of Drug–Drug Interactions

Consult your primary care doctor before taking any new drugs, including OTC drugs and dietary supplements, such as medicinal herbs. Other things that you can do include the following:

- Keep a list of all drugs being taken, and periodically discuss this list with the doctor or pharmacist.
- Keep a list of all disorders that you might have, and periodically discuss this list with the doctor.
- Select a pharmacist who provides comprehensive services (including checking for possible interactions) and who maintains a complete drug profile for each patient, and have all prescriptions dispensed by this pharmacist.
- Learn about the purpose and actions of all drugs prescribed.
- Learn about the possible side effects of the drugs.
- Learn how to take the drugs, what time of day they should be taken, and whether they can be taken during the same time period as other drugs.
- Review the use of OTC drugs with the pharmacist, and discuss any disorders that you presently have and any prescription drugs being taken.
- Take drugs as instructed on the label.
- Report to the doctor or pharmacist any symptoms that might be related to the use of a drug.
- If you are seeing more than one doctor, make sure each doctor knows all of the drugs being taken.

Foods and Drinks That Might Affect the Drugs You Are Taking

Grapefruit juice in larger quantities (8 ounces or more) can interact with the class of drugs called statins, which are used to lower lipid and cholesterol levels. Grapefruit juice is thought to block the enzyme that helps to break down the drug, so more of the drug stays

Drug–Herbal Product Interactions

in the blood longer. You should not take grapefruit juice at the same time you take statin drugs.

A drug taken alone without trouble can have a diminished effect if another drug is taken that inhibits the first drug's ability to work. An example would be tetracycline taken with an antacid containing calcium, such as TUMS. The tetracycline will have little antibiotic activity if taken at the same time as the antacid containing calcium. Dairy products consumed with tetracycline will diminish the activity of the antibiotic as well. Calcium and calcium-containing products, such as milk, cheese, and other dairy products, inhibit the action of the class of antibiotics that is made up of tetracycline and tetracycline derivatives.

Summary

In summary, please remember that it is important to recognize that any drug can interact with other drugs, herbs, or supplements. You need to check with your pharmacist if you have questions, and you always need to tell caregivers all of the drugs that you currently take.

References

Drug interactions with St. John's wort. *The Medical Letter* 2000;1081:56.

Fincham JE. Taking Your Medicine: A Guide to Medication Regimens and Compliance for Patients and Caregivers. Binghamton, NY: Pharmaceutical Products Press, Inc., 2005, pp 82–86.

The University of Michigan Health System. Selected herb-drug interactions. Available at http://www.med.umich.edu/1libr/aha/umherb01.htm; accessed March 17, 2007.

CHAPTER ELEVEN

Complementary and Alternative Medicine

Introduction

Please discuss any and all treatment options with your healthcare professional. The material presented here is for information purposes only; always check with your doctor for specific questions about your health condition.

Different Treatment Approaches

The material that is presented in this chapter may be completely new information to you. If you have received care in the healthcare system, you probably have received conventional medical treatment. Conventional medicine refers to treatments provided by allopathic physicians, such as medical doctors (MDs) or osteopathic physicians (doctor of osteopathy [DOs]), in hospitals and laboratories and in pharmacies. This is referred to as Western medical care as well. You might also have seen the care you receive termed orthodox or regular medical care.

Open-Minded View of Different Treatment Options

The material to be presented in this chapter is sometimes referred to as Eastern medicine, unorthodox, unconventional or nonconventional, unproven, or even irregular. Many of the techniques to be listed have been used for centuries and have been passed down from generation to generation. These healers and the techniques that they use can produce results and patient outcomes just as impressive as any care received elsewhere that is termed "mainstream." As you read the material, please be as open minded or as skeptical as you are when considering any form of medical treatment. I guess what I am suggesting is to look at these items in the same framework that you do when considering what might be termed orthodox medicine.

It is interesting that in parts of Asia, both Eastern and Western medicine can be presented side by side for patients to choose, and sometimes, practitioners use both approaches at the same time. For example, in Vietnam, patients can choose from traditional medicine (Eastern medicine) or Western medicine for treatments. There are facilities often in the same building side be side that can allow for these systems of care to be used in a combined fashion. The National Traditional Medicine Hospital in Hanoi is just such a facility. In the National Traditional Medicine Hospital, Western pharmaceuticals and Vietnamese traditional medicines are used together for patient treatments.

National Center for Complementary and Alternative Medicine (NCCAM)

Get the Facts

The following material is excerpted from the National Center for Complementary and Alternative Medicine Publication D-156 entitled "Get the Facts" (National Center for Complementary and Alternative Medicine, 2007). The disclaimer note that follows is provided on the site.

This publication is not copyrighted and is in the public domain. Duplication is encouraged.

NCCAM has provided this material for your information. It is not intended to substitute for the medical expertise and advice of your primary healthcare provider. We encourage you to discuss any decisions about treatment or care with your healthcare provider. The mention of any product, service, or therapy in this information is not an endorsement by NCCAM.

What is CAM?

There are many terms used to describe approaches to health care that are outside the realm of conventional medicine as practiced in the United States. This presentation explains how the National Center for Complementary and Alternative Medicine (NCCAM), a component of the

National Institutes of Health, defines some of the key terms used in the field of complementary and alternative medicine (CAM).

Complementary and alternative medicine, as defined by NCCAM, is a group of diverse medical and healthcare systems, practices, and products that are not presently considered to be part of conventional medicine. While some scientific evidence exists regarding some CAM therapies, for most there are key questions that are yet to be answered through well-designed scientific studies—questions such as whether these therapies are safe and whether they work for the diseases or medical conditions for which they are used.

The list of what is considered to be CAM changes continually, as those therapies that are proven to be safe and effective become adopted into conventional health care and as new approaches to health care emerge.

Are complementary medicine and alternative medicine different from each other?

Yes, they are different.

* **Complementary** *medicine is used* **together with** *conventional medicine. An example of a complementary therapy is using aromatherapy to help lessen a patient's discomfort following surgery.*
* **Alternative** *medicine is used* **in place of** *conventional medicine. An example of an alternative therapy is using a special diet to treat cancer instead of undergoing surgery, radiation, or chemotherapy that has been recommended by a conventional doctor.*

What is integrative medicine?

Integrative medicine, as defined by NCCAM, combines mainstream medical therapies and CAM therapies for which there is some high-quality scientific evidence of safety and effectiveness

What are the major types of complementary and alternative medicine?

NCCAM classifies CAM therapies into five categories, or domains:

1. Alternative Medical Systems

Alternative medical systems are built upon complete systems of theory and practice. Often, these systems have evolved apart from and earlier than the conventional medical approach used in the United States. Examples of alternative medical systems that have developed in Western cultures include homeopathic medicine and naturopathic medicine. Examples of systems that have developed in non-Western cultures include traditional Chinese medicine and Ayurveda.

2. *Mind-Body Interventions*

Mind-body medicine uses a variety of techniques designed to enhance the mind's capacity to affect bodily function and symptoms. Some techniques that were considered CAM in the past have become mainstream (for example, patient support groups and cognitive-behavioral therapy). Other mind-body techniques are still considered CAM, including meditation, prayer, mental healing, and therapies that use creative outlets such as art, music, or dance.

3. *Biologically Based Therapies*

Biologically based therapies in CAM use substances found in nature, such as herbs, foods, and vitamins. Some examples include dietary supplements, herbal products, and the use of other so-called natural but as yet scientifically unproven therapies (for example, using shark cartilage to treat cancer).

4. *Manipulative and Body-Based Methods*

Manipulative and body-based methods in CAM are based on manipulation and/or movement of one or more parts of the body. Some examples include chiropractic or osteopathic manipulation, and massage.

5. *Energy Therapies*

Energy therapies involve the use of energy fields. They are of two types:

• *Biofield therapies are intended to affect energy fields that purportedly surround and penetrate the human body. The existence of such fields has not yet been scientifically proven. Some forms of energy therapy manipulate biofields by applying pressure and/or manipulating the body by placing the hands in, or through, these fields. Examples include qi gong, Reiki, and Therapeutic Touch.*

• *Bioelectromagnetic-based therapies involve the unconventional use of electromagnetic fields, such as pulsed fields, magnetic fields, or alternating-current or direct-current fields.*

Conventional medicine is medicine as practiced by holders of M.D. (medical doctor) or D.O. (doctor of osteopathy) degrees and by their allied health professionals, such as physical therapists, psychologists, and registered nurses. Other terms for conventional medicine include allopathy; Western, mainstream, orthodox, and regular medicine; and biomedicine. Some conventional medical practitioners are also practitioners of CAM.

Other terms for complementary and alternative medicine include unconventional, non-conventional, unproven, and irregular medicine or health care.

Some uses of dietary supplements have been incorporated into conventional medicine. For example, scientists have found that folic acid prevents certain birth defects and that a regimen of vitamins and zinc can slow the progression of an eye disease called age-related macular degeneration (AMD).

***Acupuncture** ("AK-yoo-pungk-cher") is a method of healing developed in China at least 2,000 years ago. Today, acupuncture describes a family of procedures involving stimulation of anatomical points on the body by a variety of techniques. American practices of acupuncture incorporate medical traditions from China, Japan, Korea, and other countries. The acupuncture technique that has been most studied scientifically involves penetrating the skin with thin, solid, metallic needles that are manipulated by the hands or by electrical stimulation.*

***Aromatherapy** ("ah-roam-uh-THER-ah-py") involves the use of essential oils (extracts or essences) from flowers, herbs, and trees to promote health and well-being.*

***Ayurveda** ("ah-yur-VAY-dah") is a CAM alternative medical system that has been practiced primarily in the Indian subcontinent for 5,000 years. Ayurveda includes diet and herbal remedies and emphasizes the use of body, mind, and spirit in disease prevention and treatment.*

***Chiropractic** ("kie-roh-PRAC-tic") is a CAM alternative medical system. It focuses on the relationship between bodily structure (primarily that of the spine) and function, and how that relationship affects the preservation and restoration of health. Chiropractors use manipulative therapy as an integral treatment tool.*

***Dietary supplements.** Congress defined the term "dietary supplement" in the Dietary Supplement Health and Education Act (DSHEA) of 1994. A dietary supplement is a product (other than tobacco) taken by mouth that* *contains a "dietary ingredient" intended to supplement the diet. Dietary ingredients may include vitamins, minerals, herbs or other botanicals, amino acids, and substances such as enzymes, organ tissues, and metabolites. Dietary supplements come in many forms, including extracts, concentrates, tablets, capsules, gel caps, liquids, and powders. They have special requirements for labeling. Under DSHEA, dietary supplements are considered foods, not drugs.*

__Electromagnetic fields__ (EMFs, also called electric and magnetic fields) are invisible lines of force that surround all electrical devices. The Earth also produces EMFs; electric fields are produced when there is thunderstorm activity, and magnetic fields are believed to be produced by electric currents flowing at the Earth's core.

__Homeopathic__ ("home-ee-oh-PATH-ic") __medicine__ is a CAM alternative medical system. In homeopathic medicine, there is a belief that "like cures like," meaning that small, highly diluted quantities of medicinal substances are given to cure symptoms, when the same substances given at higher or more concentrated doses would actually cause those symptoms.

__Massage__ ("muh-SAHJ") therapists manipulate muscle and connective tissue to enhance function of those tissues and promote relaxation and well-being.

__Naturopathic__ ("nay-chur-o-PATH-ic") __medicine__, or naturopathy, is a CAM alternative medical system. Naturopathic medicine proposes that there is a healing power in the body that establishes, maintains, and restores health. Practitioners work with the patient with a goal of supporting this power, through treatments such as nutrition and lifestyle counseling, dietary supplements, medicinal plants, exercise, homeopathy, and treatments from traditional Chinese medicine

__Osteopathic__ ("ahs-tee-oh-PATH-ic") __medicine__ is a form of conventional medicine that, in part, emphasizes diseases arising in the musculoskeletal system. There is an underlying belief that all of the body's systems work together, and disturbances in one system may affect function elsewhere in the body. Some osteopathic physicians practice osteopathic manipulation, a full-body system of hands-on techniques to alleviate pain, restore function, and promote health and well-being.

__Qi gong__ ("chee-GUNG") is a component of traditional Chinese medicine that combines movement, meditation, and regulation of breathing to enhance *the flow of qi (an ancient term given to what is believed to be vital energy) in the body, improve blood circulation, and enhance immune function.*

Reiki *("RAY-kee") is a Japanese word representing Universal Life Energy. Reiki is based on the belief that when spiritual energy is channeled through a Reiki practitioner, the patient's spirit is healed, which in turn heals the physical body.*

Therapeutic Touch *is derived from an ancient technique called laying-on of hands. It is based on the premise that it is the healing force of the therapist that affects the patient's recovery; healing is promoted when the body's energies are in balance; and, by passing their hands over the patient, healers can identify energy imbalances.*

Traditional Chinese medicine (TCM) *is the current name for an ancient system of health care from China. TCM is based on a concept of balanced qi (pronounced "chee"), or vital energy, that is believed to flow throughout the body. Qi is proposed to regulate a person's spiritual, emotional, mental, and physical balance and to be influenced by the opposing forces of yin (negative energy) and yang (positive energy). Disease is proposed to result from the flow of qi being disrupted and yin and yang becoming imbalanced. Among the components of TCM are herbal and nutritional therapy, restorative physical exercises, meditation, acupuncture, and remedial massage.*

Great Sources of Further Information

A valuable resource for you to consider using is the International Bibliographic Information on Dietary Supplements (IBIDS) database; this compilation of resources on dietary supplements allows you to look up a supplement and view the research that has been carried out with the supplement (http://ods.od.nih.gov/Health_Information/IBIDS.aspx). The National Institutes of Health Office of Dietary Supplements provides this site. More information about this office is provided at the end of the following "For More Information" section.

As I noted at the start of this chapter, keep an open mind about all treatments, evaluate the risks and benefits of all treatments, and make informed decisions about which type of treatment is best for you. You doctor can provide views and opinions about your own condition and health state to guide you as well.

For More Information

NCCAM, National Institutes of Health
9000 Rockville Pike
Bethesda, Maryland 20892 USA
Web: nccam.nih.gov
E-mail: info@nccam.nih.gov

Sources of NCCAM Information

NCCAM Clearinghouse
Toll-free in the U.S.: 1-888-644-6226
International: 301-519-3153
TTY (for deaf and hard-of-hearing callers): 1-866-464-3615
E-mail: info@nccam.nih.gov
Web site: nccam.nih.gov
Address: NCCAM Clearinghouse, P.O. Box 7923, Gaithersburg, MD 20898-7923
Fax: 1-866-464-3616
Fax-on-Demand service: 1-888-644-6226

The NCCAM Clearinghouse provides information on CAM and on NCCAM. Services include fact sheets, other publications, and searches of federal databases of scientific and medical literature. The Clearinghouse does not provide medical advice, treatment recommendations, or referrals to practitioners.

Sources of Information on Dietary Supplements

Office of Dietary Supplements, NIH
Web site: ods.od.nih.gov
E-mail: ods@nih.gov

ODS supports research and disseminates research results on dietary supplements. It produces the International Bibliographic Information on Dietary Supplements (IBIDS) database on the Web, which contains abstracts of peer-reviewed scientific literature on dietary supplements.

U.S. Food and Drug Administration (FDA)
Center for Food Safety and Applied Nutrition
Web site: www.cfsan.fda.gov
Toll-free in the U.S.: 1-888-723-3366

Information includes "Tips for the Savvy Supplement User: Making Informed Decisions and Evaluating Information" (www.cfsan.fda. gov/~dms/ds-savvy.html) and updated safety information on supplements (www.cfsan.fda.gov/~dms/ds-warn.html). If you have experienced an adverse effect from a supplement, you can report it to the FDA's MedWatch program, which collects and monitors such information (1-800-FDA-1088 or www.fda.gov/medwatch).

Reference

National Center for Complementary and Alternative Medicine. Get the facts. Available at http://nccam.nih.gov/health/whatiscam/; accessed March 17, 2007.

Antibiotics

Introduction

Bacteria and viruses are everywhere. For the most part, we can survive side by side with these critters. Our immune system and natural defenses help us maintain a stable health status within and around our bodies without us being harmed. The balance of various types of bacteria in our bodies keeps bacteria and viruses in check and prevents one type of bacteria from becoming dominant and out of control. What can affect this standoff is something that changes the normal situation. Bacteria are normally present in our mouths, on our skin, in our digestive tract, and in our lungs. When the normal balance of bacteria present in us is altered, harmful bacteria can then overtake the system and lead to an infection or make us susceptible to an infection.

How Do Infections Occur?

When our resistance to infections is lowered by a weakness, infectious bacteria can then become dominant and cause us harm. This change in our normal balance of good and bad bacteria can be due to:

- A burn that damages our skin
- Exposure to a foreign type of bacteria that is not normally present
- A decrease in our immunity because of an illness, fatigue, or lack of sleep
- A high stress level
- Poor nutrition
- A virus or a fungus that alters the normal balance in our bodies

Problem of Overuse of Antibiotics

Overuse of antibiotics can alter the normal balance of bacteria in our bodies. This overuse may destroy many different types of bacteria and then lead to more infections. Overgrowth of other bacteria may result from the overuse of antibiotics. This is referred to as a secondary infection.

Hospital-Acquired Infections, or Nosocomial Infections

Hospital-acquired infections are becoming a real problem for hospitals and patients. These hospital-acquired infections are referred to as nosocomial infections. Hospital-acquired infection can affect patients admitted to the hospital for other reasons. Because of the debilitated state of the patient and the reservoir of these bacteria in the hospital, patients are much more susceptible to infection. These types of infections are termed secondary infections.

The Promise of Antibiotics

Antibiotics are the best hope we have to treat infections. Antibiotics only kill bacteria; they do not kill viruses. So if you have a common cold or other ailment caused by a virus, antibiotics will not be of any help to you and may be harmful. They can be harmful due to the fact that the beneficial bacteria may be killed by the antibiotic, leading to a more severe viral infection or another secondary infection.

History and Development of Antibiotics

The development of antibiotics is one of the great success stories of modern medicine. Antibiotics have helped us conquer bacterial infections that have devastated humankind for centuries. In 1906, a German doctor, Paul Ehrlich, coined the phrase "magic bullets." Magic bullets were prophesized to be drugs that would target specific harmful bacteria but not affect beneficial bacteria. Ehrlich became interested in using drugs to treat infections after he had a bout with tuberculosis. In 1908, Ehrlich was awarded the Nobel Prize for his theories and his research. Over the past century, we have kept in check many types of infections, only to see these infections re-emerge. Some of the infections that are back to haunt us include:

- Tuberculosis
- Types of meningitis
- Gonorrhea
- Others

127

Early Antibiotics

The modern era of antibiotic success began with the discovery of the first sulfanilamide drug by researcher Paul Gelmo in 1908. Later, in 1932, Gerhard Domagk further studied sulfa drugs as potential drugs to kill bacteria. In 1929, Sir Arthur Fleming discovered that penicillin inhibited the growth of staphylococcal bacteria. The door was now opened to the discovery of many new compounds. In the late 1930s, Selman Waksman coined the term "anti-biotic" (Latin meaning "against life") to refer to drugs that killed bacteria. From this period in the 1930s through the end of World War II, antibiotics proved to be a major modifier of battlefield deaths due to subsequent infections. Penicillin was in such short supply during World War II that the urine of soldiers treated with penicillin was strained to obtain penicillin for reuse in others.

Many drug discoveries are serendipitous, including discovering antibiotics. Melton (2005) writes, "The success of penicillin prompted an intensive search for similar compounds that could kill bacteria or stop them growing." Researchers scoured the sea, contaminated water, and earth to find other similarly successful antibiotics. Soil has proven to be a source of antibiotics as well. The antibiotic lincomycin was discovered after soil around Lincoln, Nebraska was examined for potential antibiotic drugs. A sample of dirt outside Lincoln containing *Streptomyces lincolnensis* was sent by a detail person for the Upjohn Company of Kalamazoo, Michigan to Upjohn for analysis. The rest is history so to speak.

How Do Antibiotics Work?

Some antibiotics work by preventing bacteria from multiplying and are called bacteriostatic. The erythromycin and tetracycline classes of antibiotics are bacteriostatic in nature. Other classes of drugs, such as the penicillins and cephalosporins, are termed bactericidal; they actually destroy the bacteria. Antibiotics are successful because they can target bacteria for destruction and not harm the rest of the body. Antibiotics target cell walls of bacteria; because human cells do not have cell walls, we are safe from this activity by antibiotics. There are also antibiotics to treat fungal infections. A fungus is not a bacterium, but there are drugs to treat varying fungal infections.

Bacterial Growth

Bacteria multiply countless times daily. As bacteria multiply, grow, reproduce, and expand their domain, they become more resistant to antibiotics. Bacteria may actually produce and develop a pump within themselves that pumps out toxins, such as antibiotics. Through this process of mutation, bacteria may become resistant to an antibiotic or a class of antibiotics. What we are seeing now is a rapid rise in the number of strains of bacteria that have become resistant to antibiotics that, in the past, worked very well against a bacterial strain. If the resistance is to a single type of drug, there may be other drugs within the class or in another class that will still work because the bacteria have not yet developed a resistance to them. When there is no longer any antibiotic that will work against a strain of bacteria, the issue becomes very serious.

Why are there so many newly resistant strains of bacteria to antibiotics? The reasons can include:

- Overprescribing of antibiotics by doctors
- Patients demanding that doctors write antibiotic prescriptions for them
- Prescribing antibiotics to treat viral infections
  - The most commonly occurring incidents are when antibiotics are prescribed to treat the common cold, which is caused by a viral infections

- Underuse by patients
  - Patients who do not complete the full course of antibiotics; just taking enough of the prescription until one feels better may lead to reservoirs of bacteria that then become resistant to antibiotics

Resistant Bacteria

There is a disturbing number of strains of bacteria that are termed methicillin-resistant *Staphylococcus aureus*. Methicillin is a penicillin derivate that was always the last and best resort to treat infections that simple penicillins may not have been effective against. One of these strains is a type of *Staphylococcus aureus* that has become resistant to even this powerful agent; thus we get the term methicillin-resistant *Staphylococcus aureus* (MRSA). There are still drugs that can be effective against MRSA such as vancomycin. However, this whole process of resistance is a threat to us. If you are healthy, MRSA is not as much of a concern as if you are in a debilitated state and do not have much residual immunity to fight off infections.

Vaccinations

There are vaccines available to help prevent some bacterial infections. For example, there is a vaccine for pneumonia that you should receive. If you are on Medicare and have Part B, you are eligible to receive this vaccine. Many seniors do not know about this vaccine and do not receive the shot. Please do not let another week go by without asking your doctor about this vaccine; get this vaccination as soon as possible. Your doctor can provide it for you. Pneumonia is doubly troublesome for seniors. If you develop pneumonia, see your doctor immediately. Your doctor will diagnose you and prescribe a therapy; the sooner you take antibiotics after you develop pneumonia, the better your chances are of making a full recovery.

What to Do When You Are Prescribed an Antibiotic

When prescribed an antibiotic for an infection:

- Be sure to take the full amount
- Do not save doses for later

The following guidelines are also important:

- Realize that common colds cannot be treated with antibiotics.
- We want to get better fast, but sometimes we just have to be patient and let colds run their 7-day course.
- If a cold lasts longer than 7 days, chances are you have a bacterial infection; check with your doctor!

Allergic Reactions to Antibiotics

Some individuals are allergic to one or more antibiotics. According to Consumer Reports, a small number of people will have a severe allergic reaction to antibiotics such as penicillin or other similar antibiotics (www.consumerreports.org). This type of allergic reaction usually happens within 1 hour of taking the antibiotic and can be dangerous. It happens when the body's immune system, which normally protects you against infection, overreacts to the drug. Call your doctor immediately if this happens to you.

If you have any of the following symptoms after taking an antibiotic, call your doctor immediately or go to an emergency room:

- Swelling in your throat and mouth
- Difficulty breathing
- An itchy rash (hives) on your skin; with this rash, you get white or yellow bumps and inflammation
- Feeling lightheaded or dizzy or passing out

Not everyone is allergic to antibiotics, but if you are, always let your caregivers know this at every visit! You may have an upset stomach (nausea or diarrhea) after taking an antibiotic. Ask your pharmacist if there is a way to take the drug to minimize the stomach upset. Sometimes the antibiotic will cause food to taste a little different than normal. Sometimes you may develop a minor rash when taking an antibiotic; if so:

- Call your doctor and pharmacist if you develop a rash.
- Your doctor can tell you what to do at this point.

Yeast Infections

Women can develop a yeast infection that needs to be treated after taking an antibiotic. A foul discharge from your vagina or a cheesy seepage discharge is a sign of a vaginal yeast infection. These infections can be treated with:

- A cream that is injected into your vagina with a plunger that comes with the tube of cream
- A tablet that you may take either one dose or several doses of
- A combination of the intravaginal cream and a tablet

Bladder and Kidney Infections

Sometime bladder infections go away after several days. However, see your doctor:

- If you experience painful urination
- If you have trouble urinating

If you have these symptoms, you may have a bacterial infection in your bladder or kidney and will need to take an antibiotic.

- If prescribed an antibiotic, always take the full amount unless you are experiencing a side effect.
- Remember, taking less than the full course of antibiotics can lead to bacterial resistance!

Sometimes if you have had repeat infections of your bladder or kidney:

- Your doctor may place you on an antibiotic to prevent future infections.
- The dose of the drug is often much smaller than the dose you would take for an acute infection.
- You may have to take the drug for an extended period of time.
- The benefit is that you avoid acute infections through this treatment.

Types of Infections

Table 12-1 provides a very complete listing of the various types of infections that afflict populations. This table is drawn from an internet source called Medline Plus, a service of the United States National Library of Medicine and the National Institutes of Health. The web address for this site is http://www.nlm.nih.gov/medlineplus/infections. html. Many of the infections listed have a link for accessing more information about the disease. This federal government–sponsored website is very reliable, and I would encourage you to use the site to obtain more information about the diseases listed. This is a very trustworthy site and can help in providing you with needed information. Often when we visit a doctor and are diagnosed with an infection of one type or another, we are placed on an antibiotic. Many times, we are not told much about the infection itself but just how to treat it. This informative site will provide you with information about each of the diseases listed, how they are acquired, and what can be done to treat them.

Table 12-1   Types of Infections

Abscesses

Acquired Immunodeficiency Syndrome; see AIDS

Adult Immunization; see Immunization

AIDS

AIDS and Infections

Animal Diseases and Your Health

Animal Health; see Animal Diseases and Your Health

Anthrax

Antibiotics

Antimicrobial Resistance; see Antibiotics; Infectious Diseases

Arachnoiditis; see Meningitis

Avian Influenza; see Bird Flu

Bacterial Infections

Bird Flu

Blood Poisoning; see Sepsis

Blood-Borne Pathogens; see Infection Control

Body Lice; see Parasitic Diseases

Botulinum Toxin; see Botulism

Botulism

Bronchiolitis; see Bronchitis; Respiratory Syncytial Virus Infections

Bronchitis

Bubonic Plague; see Plague

Candidiasis; see Yeast Infections

Cat Scratch Disease

Cellulitis

CFS; see Chronic Fatigue Syndrome

Clap; see Gonorrhea

CMV Infections; see Cytomegalovirus Infections

Cold, Common; see Common Cold

Common Cold

Condylomata Acuminata; see Genital Warts

Coxsackievirus Infections; see Viral Infections

Crab Lice; see Sexually Transmitted Diseases

Cryptosporidiosis

Cytomegalovirus Infections

Chagas Disease

Chickenpox

Chlamydia Infections

Chronic Bronchitis; see Bronchitis

Chronic Fatigue Syndrome

Dengue

Diphtheria

E. Coli Infections

Ebola Virus; see Hemorrhagic Fevers

EBV Infections; see Infectious Mononucleosis

Ehrlichiosis; see Tick Bites

Epstein-Barr Virus Infections; see Infectious Mononucleosis

Fever

Fifth Disease

Flu

Fungal Infections

Gastroenteritis

Genital Herpes; see Herpes Simplex

Genital Warts

German Measles; see Rubella

Germs and Hygiene

Giardia Infections

Glandular Fever; see Infectious Mononucleosis

Gonorrhea

Grippe; see Flu

Handwashing; see Germs and Hygiene

Hantavirus Infections

Head Lice

Hemorrhagic Fevers

Hepatitis

Hepatitis A

Hepatitis B

Hepatitis C

Herpes Simplex

Herpes Zoster; see Shingles

Histoplasmosis; see Fungal Infections

HIV; see AIDS

HPV

Human Immunodeficiency Virus; see AIDS

Human Papillomavirus; see HPV

Immunization

Impetigo

Infantile Paralysis; see Polio and Post-Polio Syndrome

Infection Control

Infections and Pregnancy

Infections, Bacterial; see Bacterial Infections

Infections, Fungal; see Fungal Infections

Infections, Viral; see Viral Infections

Infectious Diseases

Infectious Mononucleosis

Influenza; see Flu

Itching

Jet Lag; see Traveler's Health

Jock Itch; see Tinea Infections

Legionnaires' Disease

Leishmaniasis

Lice; see Head Lice; Parasitic Diseases

Listeria Infections

Lyme Disease

Malaria

Measles

Meningitis

Monkeypox; see Monkeypox Virus Infections

Monkeypox Virus Infections

Mononucleosis; see Infectious Mononucleosis

MRSA; see Staphylococcal Infections

Mumps

Norovirus Infections; see Gastroenteritis

Norwalk Virus Infections; see Gastroenteritis

Opportunistic Infections in AIDS; see AIDS and Infections

Paralysis, Infantile; see Polio and Post-Polio Syndrome

Parasitic Diseases

Pelvic Inflammatory Disease

Pertussis; see Whooping Cough

PID; see Pelvic Inflammatory Disease

Pinworms

Plague

Plantar Warts; see Warts

Pneumocystis Infections

Pneumonia

Polio and Post-Polio Syndrome

Post-herpetic Neuralgia; see Shingles

Pregnancy, Infections in; see Infections and Pregnancy

Q Fever; see Bacterial Infections

Rabies

Respiratory Syncytial Virus Infections

Ringworm; see Tinea Infections

Rocky Mountain Spotted Fever; see Tick Bites

Roseola; see Viral Infections

Rotavirus Infections

RSV Infections; see Respiratory Syncytial Virus Infections

Rubella

Rubeola; see Measles

Salmonella Infections

SARS; see Severe Acute Respiratory Syndrome

Scabies

Scarlet Fever; see Streptococcal Infections

Sepsis

Septic Shock; see Sepsis

Septicemia; see Sepsis

Severe Acute Respiratory Syndrome

Sexually Transmitted Diseases

Shingles

Sinusitis

Smallpox

South American Trypanosomiasis; see Chagas Disease

Staphylococcal Infections

STD; see Sexually Transmitted Diseases

Stomach Flu; see Gastroenteritis

Strep Throat; see Streptococcal Infections

Streptococcal Infections

Syphilis

TB; see Tuberculosis

Tetanus

Thrush; see Yeast Infections

Tick Bites

Tinea Infections

Toxic Shock Syndrome; see Sepsis

Toxoplasmosis

Traveler's Health

Trichomoniasis

Tropical Medicine; see Traveler's Health

Tuberculosis

Tularemia; see Tick Bites

Universal Precautions; see Infection Control

Vaccination; see Immunization

Varicella-Zoster Virus; see Chickenpox

Venereal Disease; see Sexually Transmitted Diseases

Viral Hepatitis; see Hepatitis

Viral Infections

Warts

West Nile Virus

Whooping Cough

Yeast Infections

Yellow Fever; see Viral Infections

Zoonoses; see Animal Diseases and Your Health

Antibiotics

Source: Medline Plus, A service of the United States National Library of Medicine and the National Institutes of Health. Infections. Available at http://www.nlm.nih.gov/medlineplus/infections.html; accessed January 27, 2007.

For More Information

For a great resource on infections, both in general and for specific infections, go to the following Medline Plus website: http://www.nlm. nih.gov/medlineplus/infections.html.

Reference

Melton L. Drugs in peril: How do antibiotics work? Welcome Trust, July 1, 2005. Available at http://www.wellcome.ac.uk/doc_WTX026109.html; accessed January 25, 2007.

CHAPTER THIRTEEN

Resources Available to Help You with Medicare Part D

Introduction

The coverage of prescription drugs in the Medicare program is a major change in the insurance available for health care for seniors. Since 1965 when Medicare was enacted, seniors have faced many dilemmas when choosing to purchase prescription drugs. Until now, you had to pay for drugs on your own or through other insurance policies. Now, you can receive help with the cost of your prescription drugs in the new Medicare Part D.

Medicare Part D: A Complex Program

Many aspects of this program are hard to understand. Formularies, provider status, copayments, deductibles, and petitions for service are several confusing elements of Medicare Part D. The Part D program will no doubt change in the coming months and subsequent years. The more you can do to educate yourself about the benefit now will help you in the coming months and beyond.

You may be eligible for extra coverage under Medicare Part D. You will want to choose a program that allows you to continue to take the drugs you are taking now and at the lowest cost available. It will take some time for you to figure this out, but you can easily do this. You may need to have someone help you, but the extra effort expended at the start of your seeking a plan will help you later on. If you can use a computer or have a friend or family member who can use a computer, this will be a big help to you in the decision-making process.

Prescription Drug Plans

Much of the information available for the Medicare Part D program is online at the following website: www.medicare.gov. This site provides information on the various options available to you to consider for your choice of a Medicare Part D drug plan. The plans available are what are called stand-alone prescription drug plans. The only services they provide are for prescription drugs.

Medicare Advantage Plans

There is another option for you to consider. This option is called a Medicare Advantage Plan. The Medicare Advantage option is one of two types of prescription drug plans in Medicare Part D. Medicare Advantage Plans are health plan options that are part of the Medicare program. If you join one of these plans, you generally get all of your Medicare-covered health care through that plan. This coverage can include *prescription drug coverage*. Medicare Advantage Plans include:

- Medicare Health Maintenance Organization (HMOs)
- Preferred Provider Organizations (PPO)
- Private Fee-for-Service Plans
- Medicare Special Needs Plans

When you join a Medicare Advantage Plan, you use the health insurance card that you get from the plan for your health care. In most of these plans, generally, there are extra benefits and lower copayments than in the original Medicare Plan. However, you may have to see doctors who belong to the plan or go to certain hospitals or pharmacies to obtain services.

Managed Care

HMOs and PPOs are a type of insurance called managed care. In these plans, you obtain care from select providers that the HMO or PPO works with. You may not be able to use doctors outside of these plans without paying extra. Please see Table 13-1 for a listing of the various types of Medicare insurance. This table describes the various parts of Medicare (A, B, C, D) and indicates what services are provided in each of the Medicare parts. One thing to remember is that you must have signed up for Medicare Part A and Part B in order to obtain prescription drug coverage under Medicare Part D.

Table 13-1   Medicare Insurance Program

Medicare Part	What Does It Cover?	What Types of Services Are Included?	Do You Need to Sign Up for the Plan?
Part A	Hospital Insurance	Inpatient hospital services, skilled nursing facilities, home care	No need to sign up; you are automatically eligible at age 65; payroll taxes finance the plan, so you pay no premiums
Part B	Supplemental Medical Insurance	Physician and other health care provider office visits, outpatient services, drugs administered in an outpatient clinic	Pay by premiums, which vary per month, and the rates are raised each year; you must sign up for Part B Medicare
Medicare Advantage	Medicare Advantage (managed care) Formerly Medicare+Choice, or Medicare Part C	Medicare Parts A, B, and D provided through a private health plan such as a managed care organization (HMO)	You sign up for Medicare Advantage, and it is paid for by a combination of payroll taxes and premiums
Part D	Prescription Drug Insurance	Outpatient prescription drugs such as those purchased in a community pharmacy or from an outpatient hospital pharmacy	Premiums vary depending upon which plan you choose

What You Should Know before Signing Up for Medicare Part D Coverage

Are Your Drugs Covered?

This question is really important for you to spend time considering. The issue is that all of the drugs that you take now may not be covered in a plan that you might choose. This means that you will have to pay for the drug out of your own pocket if you choose a particular plan without coverage for your drug. A recent study conducted by the Kaiser Family Foundation concluded that, on average, 80% of a listing of commonly used drugs was covered under most plans participating in Medicare Part D. No plan covered all of the drugs, and the range of coverage was from 64% to 97%. Most plans operate with what is termed a tiered coverage scheme. The tiers are differing types of drugs for which you will pay different amounts of copayment or cost-sharing amounts.

One of the parts of this new Medicare Part D is what is called a formulary. Part of this formulary coverage for your drugs is a "tiering" system of different prices for drugs that you might be taking. You will pay less for a generic drug (tier 1) than you will for what is called a preferred brand name drug (tier 2), and you will pay the most for a brand name drug (tier 3). This third tier is for brand name drugs that are called nonpreferred. Please see Table 13-2 for a depiction of what a drug tier looks like. The amounts listed under Amount to Pay in this table are for illustrative purposes only. The actual amounts that you will pay will vary from prescription drug plan to prescription drug plan.

What Pharmacies Can I Use to Obtain My Prescriptions?

To provide as much coverage as possible, many pharmacies can fill your prescriptions under this benefit. However, not all pharmacies may be in the network (the listing of pharmacies eligible to be used in your prescription plan), so you may not be able to use your normal pharmacy. This is something that you should check on before you sign up for a plan. Many pharmacies belong to many networks and thus can fill your prescriptions; others may not be able to.

Table 13-2   Example of a Tiered Arrangement for a Type of Drug

Tier	Drugs Covered	Amount to Pay
First Tier	A generically available drug (generic)	$ 5.00
Second Tier	A preferred brand name drug	$25.00
Third Tier	A nonpreferred brand name drug	$60.00

How Do I Sign Up?

Please know that even if you are eligible to sign up for Medicare Part D, you may choose not to sign up for coverage. However, if you do not do so in the time period allotted, you will have to pay an additional amount per month (a 1% penalty) plus the regular amount of the monthly premium. It is also important for you to know that, once you sign up for a particular plan, you must stay with this plan for the balance of the year. However, if you are dissatisfied with the plan that you originally signed up for, you can change to a different plan for the next year.

What Do I Need to Know to Get Started?

So what do you need to know to get started? There are several key things that you need to know to obtain the most from this benefit.

- Know your drugs; what are the drugs you take and what are their complete names?
- Know your pharmacist; will the pharmacy you use be able to continue to take care of your needs?
- Know which of your drugs are available as generic substitutes; have your pharmacist help you with this.
- Use as many generic drugs as you can.
  - This will be a key way to save money with this program.
- Know approximately how much you will spend for drugs per year; your pharmacist can help you with this.
- Know as much as you can about the Medicare Part D benefits. Do you know how to make these benefits work for you?
- Know what the "donut hole" gap in coverage means to you and how to make sure that you can diminish its impact on your costs.
- Know who can help you with understanding this program and its components.

Caution About Scam Artists

I want you to be extra cautious about scam artists who may try to take advantage of you! If someone tries to sell you insurance and asks for bank information, they are not to be trusted. Likewise, if someone claims that you can obtain a new Medicare insurance card for an amount of money, they too are trying to take advantage of you. So, please be cautious about those from whom you seek information or insurance coverage. Nowhere are people immune from these scams. In July of 2004, it was reported that fraudulent contacts were made in many large and smaller communities in Nebraska. Nebraska state officials and other agencies had received complaints. In this scam, callers identified themselves as representing nonexistent but legitimate-sounding groups. The callers offer to help seniors with the difficult Medicare Part D program. The callers then asked for money or credit card numbers to provide service to individuals. No legitimate Medicare Part D plan will ask for money or credit card information over the phone.

Prescription Drug Plans

Prescription drug plans (PDPs) are free-standing plans that will provide services on a fee-for-service basis. This means that you pay for your medications as you always do until you reach a certain amount paid. This amount is called a deductible. As you start the coverage with this plan, you will pay for your prescriptions until you reach the deductible amount (for example, $265 in 2007). Some plans do not have a deductible. This is done in order to get as many people as possible to sign up for the coverage. So there is a trade-off that you have to consider; you may pay a little more for a monthly premium but not have to pay any deductible. You might also have coverage in the so-called "donut hole" and have coverage for your drugs throughout the year. So, it is really important to consider all of these facts when you decide on a plan. Also, realize that, although you are tied to a plan for the balance of the year once you sign up, you can switch plans for the next year. So a plan that does not meet all of your needs one year can be dropped for another plan the next year.

There are several things to consider concerning the PDPs and the differences between them. Each plan will provide an overview of important information about each PDP, how much the monthly premiums are, what the PDP will pay for and what it covers, and whether the PDP offers a mail service prescription option. On the Medicare website and in their written materials, there are numerous points that you can consider.

Medicare Advantage Plans

The second type of prescription plan that will be available to you is what is termed a Medicare Advantage plan. There are several things that you can decide on concerning the Medicare Advantage Plans and the differences between them. Each plan will provide an overview of important information and information on how much the monthly premiums are and what the Medicare Advantage plan will pay for and what it covers. On the Medicare website and in their written materials, there are numerous points that you can consider.

Network Pharmacy

Like the prescription drug plans (PDPs), each Medicare Advantage Part D drug plan has a network of pharmacies for members to use to fill prescriptions. This network may be national in scope and include many pharmacies across the state where you live and across the nation. Others may have a much smaller network of eligible pharmacies for you to use. This is information that is available from each plan. The best way to find the answer to the question of which pharmacies can be used is to ask your pharmacist where you obtain your current prescriptions. He or she will easily be able to advise you as to whether you have many pharmacies to choose from or a much smaller number of potential pharmacies at which to obtain your medications.

Coverage of Classes of Drugs

One aspect of the Medicare Part D Program that Medicare officials have put in place is ensuring that certain drugs are covered. This is the case no matter whether you have a prescription drug plan or a Medicare Advantage plan. This is only fair and is a very nice component of this new plan. Basically, Medicare officials did not want anyone to be slighted in this new plan. So to protect against discrimination, the Centers for Medicare and Medicaid Services (CMS) has reviewed six drug classes (types of drugs to treat the same condition) and made the stipulation that certain drugs will be covered. These drug classes include the following:

- Antidepressants
  - Drug to treat depression
- Antipsychotics
  - Drugs to treat certain mental disorders
- Anticonvulsants
  - Drugs to control seizures
- Antiretrovirals
  - Drugs for patients with acquired immunodeficiency syndrome (AIDS) and HIV
- Antineoplastics
  - Drugs to treat cancer of one type or another
- Immunosuppressants
  - Drugs that are prescribed when a patient has had an organ transplantation; these drugs work to stop the problem of organ rejection

Learning about Different Plans

You will need to spend time examining what options are available to you in your region of the country. There are several options available to you. I encourage you to have someone help you at this point. You will need to know the exact spelling of the drugs that you take. Know whether you take a once-daily drug that has an extended-release form. The XL, SR, and CR letters that follow the names of your drugs are very important for you to know. Some plans might cover some of the forms of the drug that you take, but they may not cover the exact formulation that you take. Keep looking until you can determine whether the plan you choose will cover your present drugs. On some prescription containers, there are only abbreviated spellings of the drug names. It is important for you to know the complete names of the drugs you take.

Know When You Need to Sign Up for Coverage

Be sure to know the times of the year when you are eligible to sign up for coverage. Also, be aware that the plans available in 2008 for your consideration will be available for review in October 2007.

Where Can You Apply?

There are several places where you can apply for extra help coverage:

- At your local Social Security office (the Social Security Administration [SSA] will also take an application over phone)
- Through your state Medicaid office
- Through programs called state health insurance assistance programs (SHIPs)
- Through the SSA website (www.ssa.gov/prescriptionhelp)

How Do I Find Out Whether I Qualify for Extra Help?

You may qualify for extra help if you have limited income and resources. Limited income, as of August 2006 (this may change in the future as adjustments are made), is $14,700 or less for a single individual and $19,800 or less for a married couple. If your income is higher, you may still qualify for extra help, for example, if you support family members who live with you or you have some earnings from a job. Also, if you live in Alaska or Hawaii, these income limits are different, so you may qualify if your income is higher.

You may also receive help from other sources. These additional means of support do not count as part of your income! They should not be entered in the total for your income estimate. These other sources of support include:

- Food stamp assistance
- Home energy assistance
- Housing assistance
- Disaster assistance (help during Hurricane Katrina, for example)
- Earned income tax credits
- Victim compensation
- Scholarships and/or educational grants

When you are filling out the required forms, limited resources refers to less than $10,000 for an individual or less than $20,000 for a married couple. You can also add an extra $1,500 per person if you will use funds for burial purposes. Please note that the following do not count as resources:

- Your primary residence
- Your personal possessions
- Your vehicles
- Items like jewelry or home furnishings—things you could not easily convert to cash
- Rental property that you need for self-support; this might include land that you use to grow produce for home consumption
- Nonbusiness property that is essential for your self-sufficiency
- Cash life insurance policies of up to $1,500 for singles and $3,000 for couples living together
- Burial plots

If you have Medicaid prescription benefits, your costs will be greatly reduced in Medicare Part D.

Should I Sign Up for Medicare Part D?

Please see Figure 13-1 for a decision tree you can use to help you make decisions about Medicare Part D.

CREDITABLE COVERAGE

Creditable coverage is coverage that you currently have from other plans that is as good as or better than the Medicare plans that are available to you. If you have such a plan that is provided to you by an employer, or former employer, and it is a good plan, you should not sign up for the Medicare Part D program. If you sign up for coverage under Medicare Part D, you will be assessed a penalty each month plus the normal monthly premium.

THERE ARE CONSEQUENCES IF YOU DO NOT SIGN UP WHEN YOU ARE ELIGIBLE

There are consequences if you do not sign up when you are eligible. For example, what if you did not enroll in a Medicare prescription drug plan by May 15, 2006, which was the end of the Initial Enrollment Period (IEP)? You do not have creditable coverage and you wait to enroll in a prescription Part D drug plan in November 2006, during the Annual Coordinated Election Period. The penalty will be 6% because you had 6 months without creditable coverage, starting with the first month you would have been covered if you had joined a plan by May 15. So, count the months of June, July, August, September, October, and November. Since the base national premium in 2007 was $27.35 per month, then your penalty would be $27.35 × 0.06 = $1.64 per month. This will be added to the premium payment amount. It is calculated by multiplying 1% of the base beneficiary premium by the number of months the person was eligible but not enrolled in a plan and did not have creditable drug coverage. The penalty calculation is not based on the premium of the plan the individual is enrolled in. The base beneficiary premium is a national number and can change each year.

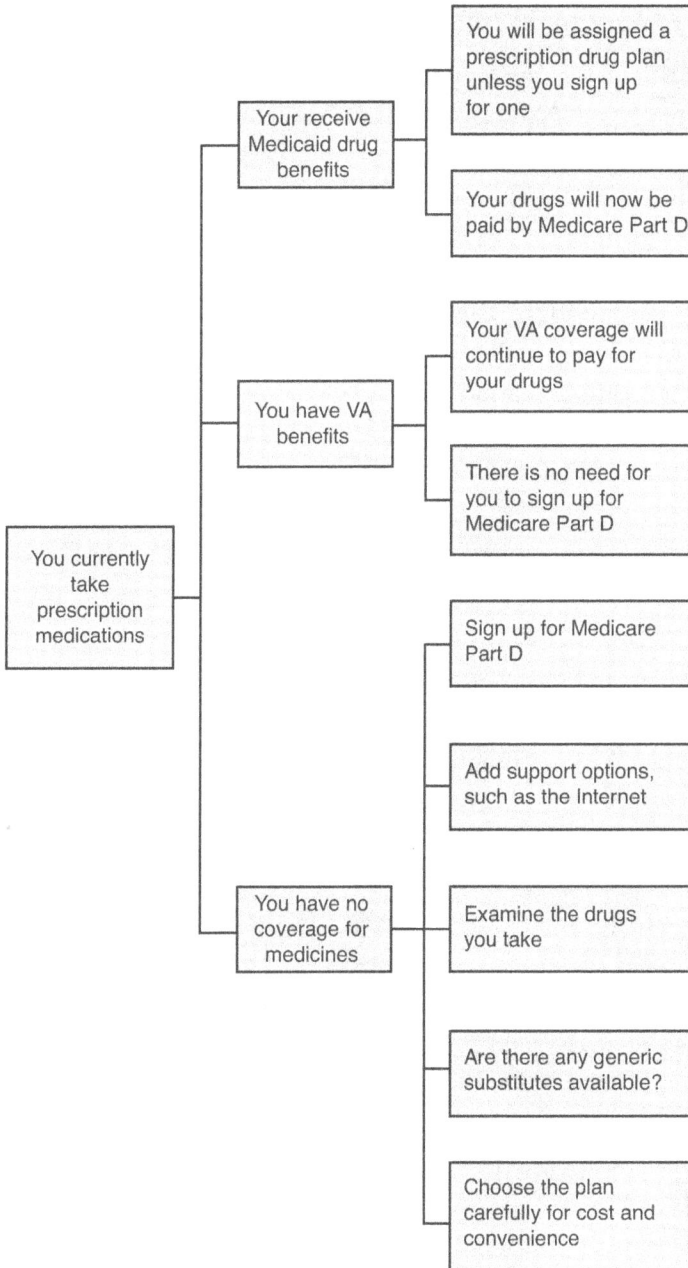

Figure 13-1   Decisions about Medicare Part D.

What Happens When People First become Eligible to Enroll in a Medicare Drug Plan?

All people who become entitled to Medicare after January 2006 have a 7-month Initial Enrollment Period (IEP) for enrollment in Part D:

- They can apply 3 months before their month of Medicare eligibility. Coverage will begin on the date they become eligible.
- They can apply in their month of eligibility, in which case their Part D coverage will begin on the first of the following month.
- Or they can also apply during the 3 months after their month of eligibility, with coverage beginning on the first of the month after the month in which they apply.

Some groups of people who become entitled to Medicare will be enrolled in a Part D plan by CMS unless they join a plan on their own.

How Can I Pay for My Premiums?

You can pay for your premiums in several ways, including the following:

- You can mail monthly premium payments to the plan you sign up with
- You can automatically transfer the premium for your plan from your bank accounts, either checking or savings
- You can also have monthly premiums taken out of your monthly Social Security benefit

As is the case with many types of withdrawals, it will take time (a couple of months, depending on what time of the month you sign up) before the Social Security deduction is in effect. The way this works is that 2 months of your premiums are taken out with the first payment made, and then single payments will be deducted thereafter. If you enroll in December of the year, you will probably be billed in

February for both the January and February premiums. This is a government program, and it may take 3 or more months for this to be put in place! If it is more than 3 months, you will be contacted to see how you want your premiums deducted.

Drugs That Are Not Covered

There are several types of drugs that are not available for coverage in the Medicare Part D program. These drug classes include:

- Over-the-counter drugs
- Barbiturates
- Benzodiazepines
- Vitamins
- Drugs to lose weight
- Drugs for cosmetic purposes
- Drugs for erectile dysfunction

It does not matter if your doctor has written you prescriptions for these drugs. They are not covered under Medicare Part D.

Formularies

A list of drugs that a Medicare drug plan covers is called a formulary. Formularies include generic drugs and brand name drugs. Most prescription drugs used by people with Medicare will be on a plan's formulary. The formulary must include at least two drugs in the categories and classes of drugs most commonly prescribed to people with Medicare. This makes sure that people with different medical conditions can get the treatment they need.

Not all formularies are the same. Some drug plans may cover more drugs than others.

OTHER SPECIFIC FORMULARY ISSUES

There are several things that may be required before you can be prescribed certain drugs within the Part D program. These need to be explained. They include:

- Step therapy
- Prior authorization
- Preferred drug lists
- Tiered copayments
- Pharmacy networks
- Dispensing limits

Step Therapy

Step therapy occurs when you have to try one medication and see whether it works for your condition before trying a more expensive drug. In the case of blood pressure medications, there may be an older drug that must be tried before a newer drug can be prescribed. The goal of step therapies is to have a person try one medication on a short-term basis (usually a less expensive drug) before a newer and more expensive drug is prescribed. You should look at the drug plan that you choose carefully. Examine what the policy is regarding step therapy and the associated requirements.

Prior Authorization

Prior authorization is a requirement that the drug plan must approve the use of a particular drug before your doctor can prescribe it for you. The drug in question may be an expensive drug. There may also be less expensive alternatives that may be equally effective. The plan that you choose will spell out what the policy is regarding prior authorization.

Preferred Drug Lists

Prescription drug plans may have listings of drugs that are referred to as preferred drug lists. For drugs on this list, your copayment, if you are required to pay a copayment, may be less than the amount that you have to pay if a drug is not on this list. If your doctor disagrees with this, you can petition to have the drug paid for with the same copayment as the preferred drugs. So, you may have to pay a varying amount of a copayment depending on whether the drug is classified as preferred or nonpreferred by the drug plan. If you qualify for extra help under Medicare Part D, this varying copayment may not affect you at all.

Tiered Copayments

Tiered copayments refer to different amounts that you would pay as a copayment. Tiered copayments work as follows. If you are taking a generic medication, your copayment would be the lowest. Next, you may pay a higher copayment for a preferred drug (see previous section). Then, if you use a brand name drug, you will pay a higher copayment than you would pay for both generic and preferred drugs. Finally, if you are prescribed a drug for a condition for which the drug has not been approved, you may be required to pay the entire amount for the prescription. Doctors may prescribe a drug for any reason, even if the drug has not been approved to treat the condition that you have. This is called "off-label" prescribing. You should know whether you are taking any drugs for an off-label purpose; ask your doctor. If you are taking off-label drugs, then perhaps you can be prescribed another drug on a lower tier for which you can pay a lower copayment.

Pharmacy Networks

Some of the Medicare Part D drug plans or Medicare Advantage plans may limit the places where you can obtain your prescriptions. I would advise you to check with your pharmacist before you sign up for a plan to see whether or not you can continue to use that particular pharmacy for your prescription needs. Having said this, many pharmacies will participate in all of the drug plans available to them. Many of the national chain community pharmacies or supermarket pharmacies are in this category. They provide national coverage for your needs.

Dispensing Limits

Your prescription drug plan may limit the amount of a prescription that you can obtain. You may be restricted to a 30-day supply of the medications, even if you take the drug every day and will do so for a long period of time. There might be a mail order option with your drug plan, and if so, you may be able to obtain larger amounts of the prescription if you use this mail order option. This will vary from plan to plan. If this is an important issue for you, be sure to ask about this before you sign up for a prescription drug plan. Not all formularies are the same. Some drug plans may cover more drugs than others.

USE OF GENERIC DRUGS

Generic drugs will save you money. They will be less expensive than preferred drugs, brand name drugs, and drugs that your doctor may prescribe off-label. Off-label means prescribed for a reason other than normal use.

Summary

There has been a lot of information presented in this chapter. There are some basic issues that you need to decide upon. Here is a list of the basics that you need to consider:

- *Cost*—This includes the premium amount, the deductible, and the copayments required before higher levels of support kick in for you. Copayments may be different for generic drugs, brand name drugs, and other brand name preferred drugs. There is a need for you to consider many factors presented in this book.
- *Formulary coverage*—This coverage will vary from plan to plan. Your drugs may not be covered in each of the plans. The formulary finder will allow you to see what is available in your state and how many of your drugs are covered. The nice thing about the formulary finder that CMS provides is that it allows you to see whether generic drugs are available for the drugs that you are required to take.

- *Coverage gap*—There is a coverage gap that some of you will need to consider. Some plans provide some coverage for the drugs that you take in this gap ("donut hole"). Here, your true out of pocket (TrOOP) costs come into play.

- *Convenience*—Can you obtain your medicines at your regular pharmacy? This is an important issue for many people. Check to see whether your pharmacy participates in one or more of the plans that you are considering.

- *Peace of mind*—It may be to your benefit to sign up for a plan. You never know how many drugs you might have to take in the future.

- *Creditable coverage*—Determine whether the coverage that you have now is better than what you might have with the Medicare Part D plan. Remember, if you lose your creditable coverage for a reason out of your control, you will qualify for signing up for Medicare Part D. If you have Medigap prescription coverage from a company, generally, this will not be as good as what you can obtain through the Medicare Part D program.

- *If you move*, you will have up to 4 months to select a new plan. However, you must notify the plan that you currently have that you are moving to a different permanent address.

- *If you are not satisfied with your current Medicare Part D prescription drug plan*, please know that you can change plans during the next enrollment period. Outside of this enrollment period, it will be difficult for you to change plans. If you qualify for extra help, you will be able to switch plans.

Consider all of these points, think about what is best for you, and please make the most informed decision that you can. You owe it to yourself to get the most from all of the Medicare programs you participate in, including this new Medicare Part D plan.

Reference

Fincham J. The Medicare Part D Drug Program: Making the Most of the Benefit. Sudbury, MA: Jones and Bartlett, 2007.

CHAPTER FOURTEEN

Other Resources to Help You with Medicare

Introduction

The material in this chapter is meant to inform you about other services that are now available for Medicare recipients. This information has been available since July of 2006 and has been provided in various forms during training sessions sponsored by the Centers for Medicare and Medicaid Services (CMS). As is the case with all aspects of Medicare, things can change with the program, so please know that you might have to check with CMS (www.medicare.gov) about the specific details of these programs.

Medicare and Preventive Services

Medicare is focusing on preventive health more than ever before. Preventive services are things that you can do to help yourself stay as healthy as possible.

Preventive services:

- Help you to achieve the best health possible with your health conditions
- Help to keep you out of hospitals and nursing homes
- Include health screenings and vaccinations for influenza (flu shots), hepatitis B, and pneumonia

The best way to stay healthy is to live a healthy lifestyle. You can live a healthy lifestyle by exercising, eating well, keeping a healthy weight, and not smoking. Another important way to stay healthy is to get disease prevention and early detection services. These services can detect health problems early when treatment works best and can keep you from getting certain diseases or illnesses.

Many people with Medicare do not take full advantage of their Medicare-covered preventive benefits. For example:

- All people with Medicare can get a flu shot, but only 73% did so during the 2003–2004 flu season

- Medicare pays for annual mammograms, but only about 50% of eligible women had one in 2003
- Medicare also covers a variety of tests to detect colon cancer, but less than half of the people with Medicare have taken advantage of this important benefit

Talk with your doctor or healthcare provider to find out what preventive services you need and how often you need them to stay healthy. Medicare coverage of these services is based on your age, whether you are male or female, and your medical history. You must have Part B of Medicare to have these services covered.

The services in the following list are covered no matter what kind of Medicare health plan you have. However, the rules for how much you pay for these services may vary. Preventive services included in the Medicare benefit are as follows:

- "Welcome to Medicare" physical exam
  - This might also be a "brown bag" review of your medicines by a pharmacist in a formal educational format.
- Bone mass measurement
- Cardiovascular screening
- Colorectal cancer screening
- Diabetes screening, services (including diabetes self-management training and medical nutrition therapy), and supplies
- Glaucoma screening
- Pap test and pelvic examination with clinic breast examination
- Prostate cancer screening
- Screening mammogram
- Help with quitting smoking and tobacco use
- Vaccinations (shots) for:
  - Flu
  - Pneumococcal pneumonia
  - Hepatitis B

In 2007, Medicare added:

- Ultrasound screening coverage for abdominal aortic aneurysms (based on a referral from the "Welcome to Medicare" physical exam) with no deductible. The aorta is the largest artery in your body, and it carries blood away from your heart. When it reaches your abdomen, it is called the abdominal aorta. The abdominal aorta supplies blood to the lower part of the body. Just below the abdomen, the aorta splits into two branches that carry blood into each leg. When a weak area of the abdominal aorta expands or bulges, it is called an abdominal aortic aneurysm.
- No deductible for colorectal cancer screening in the Original Medicare Plan.

More Information about the "Welcome to Medicare" Physical Exam

Medicare covers a one-time preventive physical exam **within the first 6 months you have Part B**. The exam includes a thorough review of your health; education and counseling about the preventive services you need, like certain screenings and shots; and referrals for other care if you need it. The "Welcome to Medicare" physical exam is a great way to get up to date on important screenings and shots and to talk with your doctor about your family history and how to stay healthy. As previously mentioned, this "Welcome to Medicare" physical might include a comprehensive "brown bag" review of your medications to check for appropriateness of your drug therapy.

In the Original Medicare Plan, you generally pay 20% of the Medicare-approved amount after the yearly Part B deductible. (As mentioned earlier, you may have to pay copayments for preventive services if you are in a Medicare Advantage Plan or other Medicare plan.) The "Welcome to Medicare" physical exam is only available to people whose Part B coverage began on or after January 1, 2005.

If you have a standardized Medicare supplement policy, or Medigap, that policy will pay the 20%. If you have another type of healthcare coverage (such as a plan from your former employer), that policy may pay the 20%.

For each service mentioned in this chapter, I will note the cost for people in the Original Medicare Plan to get the service from a doctor or other healthcare provider who participates in Medicare and who accepts assignment. (This means that the provider will accept the Medicare-approved amount as payment in full.) However, please remember that if you get the service from a doctor who does not participate in Medicare or who does not accept assignment, you may be responsible for a higher amount. If you are in a Medicare Advantage Plan or other Medicare plan and get Medicare-covered preventive services, you may have copayments.

Preventive Services

OSTEOPOROSIS

Medicare covers bone mass measurement for certain people at risk for osteoporosis. Osteoporosis is a disease in which your bones become weak. In general, the lower your bone mass (density), the higher your risk is for a fracture (broken bone). Bone mass measurement test results will help you and your doctor choose the best way to keep your bones strong.

How often is it covered?

• Once every 24 months

Who is covered?

• Certain people with Medicare who are at risk for osteoporosis are eligible. Other people who have been diagnosed with osteoporosis or related conditions are also covered for this test and may be tested more frequently.

What are your costs in the Original Medicare Plan?

- You pay 20% of the Medicare-approved amount after the yearly Part B deductible.

Your risk for osteoporosis increases if you:

- Are age 50 or older
- Are a woman
- Have a family history or personal history of broken bones
- Are white or Asian
- Are small boned
- Have low body weight (less than approximately 127 pounds)
- Smoke and/or drink a lot of alcohol
- Have a low-calcium diet

CARDIOVASCULAR SCREENING

Medicare covers cardiovascular screening tests that check your cholesterol and other blood fat (lipid) levels. High levels of cholesterol can increase your risk for heart disease and stroke. These screenings will determine whether you have high cholesterol. You might be able to make lifestyle changes (like changing your diet) to lower your cholesterol.

What is covered?

- Tests for cholesterol, lipid, and triglyceride levels

How often are these tests covered?

- Medicare will cover these tests every 5 years.

Who is covered?

- All people with Medicare who have no apparent signs or symptoms of cardiovascular disease are eligible.

What are your costs in the Original Medicare Plan?

- You pay nothing. This is an added incentive for people to use this benefit.

COLORECTAL CANCER

Colorectal cancer is usually found in people age 50 or older, and the risk of getting colorectal cancer increases with age. Medicare covers colorectal screening tests for all people with Medicare aged 50 and older. These tests help detect cancer and find precancerous polyps (growths in the colon) so they can be removed before they turn into cancer. Treatment works best when colorectal cancer is found early. A **fecal occult blood test** is a test for blood in the stool. The patient places stool samples on a card and returns it to the doctor. This test is covered once every 12 months. A **flexible sigmoidoscopy** is a procedure that uses a thin, flexible, lighted tube to examine the lining of the rectum and lower part of the colon. The procedure is covered once every 48 months. A **screening colonoscopy** is a procedure that examines the lining of the rectum and entire colon using a thin, flexible, lighted tube to find and remove most polyps and some cancers. It is covered once every 24 months if you are at high risk for colon cancer. If you are not at high risk for colon cancer, it is covered once every 10 years but not within 48 months of a screening flexible sigmoidoscopy. There is no minimum age for colonoscopy if you are at high risk for colon cancer. You are at **high risk** if you have had or have a close relative who has had colorectal polyps or colorectal cancer or if you have inflammatory bowel disease. A **barium enema** is a procedure that allows the doctor to see an x-ray image of the rectum and entire colon. Your doctor may order this test as a substitute for a sigmoidoscopy or colonoscopy.

Payment rates vary with the type of test. In the Original Medicare Plan, you pay nothing for the fecal occult blood test. For all other tests, you pay 20% of the Medicare-approved amount after the annual Part B deductible. For flexible sigmoidoscopy or colonoscopy, you pay 25% of the Medicare-approved amount if the test is done in a hospital outpatient department. As of January 1, 2007, there is no deductible for colorectal cancer screenings.

DIABETES

Diabetes is a disease in which the body does not produce or properly use **insulin**. Insulin is a hormone that is needed to change sugar, starch, and other food into energy needed for daily life. Proper control of blood sugar can avoid or delay the complications of diabetes. Diabetes can affect many parts of the body and can lead to serious complications such as blindness, kidney damage, and lower limb amputations. You can manage your diabetes by:

- Testing your blood sugar regularly
- Eating a proper diet
- Exercising regularly
- Taking the medications your doctor prescribes (see the following website: www.diabetes.org/about-diabetes.jsp)

Medicare pays for diabetes screening tests for the purpose of early detection of diabetes in people at risk. The diabetes screening test includes a fasting blood glucose test.

Talk with your doctor about how often you should get tested. For people with prediabetes, Medicare covers a maximum of two diabetes screening tests within a 12-month period (but not less than 6 months apart). For those who are not diabetics or have not been diagnosed as prediabetics, Medicare covers one diabetes screening test within a 12-month period. You will not be responsible for a deductible or copayment in the Original Medicare Plan. Persons may be considered at high risk for diabetes if they have any of the following risk factors:

- High blood pressure
- High blood cholesterol
- Obesity
- History of high blood sugar
- At least two of the following characteristics:
  - 65 years of age or older
  - Overweight (body mass index greater than 25 but less than 30 kg/m2)
  - Family history of diabetes
  - History of gestational diabetes mellitus or delivery of a baby weighing more than 9 lbs

What Is Covered?

Medicare covers diabetes screenings for **all people with Medicare who are at risk for diabetes**. For **people with diabetes**, Medicare covers certain services and supplies to treat diabetes and help prevent its complications. In most cases, your doctor must write an order or referral for you to get these services. These services include diabetes self-management training and medical nutrition therapy, under certain conditions. Medicare will also pay for diabetic supplies, including blood sugar monitors, lancets, and testing strips, whether or not you are insulin dependent. Insulin and supplies used to inject it are covered under Medicare's prescription drug coverage. For people with diabetes, Medicare also covers hemoglobin A1c tests (a blood test to measure how well your blood sugar has been controlled over the past 3 months) and special eye exams.

Medicare also covers insulin pumps, special foot care, and therapeutic shoes for people with diabetes who need them. So, what do you have to pay? In the Original Medicare Plan, you pay 20% of the Medicare-approved amount after the annual Part B deductible for diabetes training, a monitor, lancets, and test strips, as well as medical nutrition therapy. For more information, get a free copy of *Medicare Coverage of Diabetes Supplies & Services* (CMS Publication 11022) at www.medicare.gov.

GLAUCOMA

Glaucoma is an eye disease caused by above-normal pressure in the eye. It usually damages the optic nerve, and you may gradually lose sight without symptoms. It can result in blindness, especially without treatment. The best way for people at high risk for glaucoma to protect themselves is to have regular eye exams. A glaucoma screening is an eye exam used to detect glaucoma. Medicare provides annual coverage for glaucoma screening for people with Medicare in the following high-risk categories:

- Individuals with diabetes
- Individuals with a family history of glaucoma

- African-Americans age 50 and over
- Beginning on January 1, 2006, the high-risk category was expanded to include Hispanic-Americans age 65 and over

Glaucoma exams are covered once every 12 months. You pay 20% of the Medicare-approved amount after the Part B yearly deductible in the Original Medicare Plan.

PAP TEST

Another preventive service, for women only, is a screening Pap test and pelvic exam with clinical breast examination. The Pap test is used to help find cervical and vaginal cancer. The screening pelvic exam is used to help find fibroids or ovarian cancers. As part of the pelvic exam, Medicare covers a clinical breast exam to check for breast cancer. A clinical breast exam is another way, in addition to mammograms, to look for breast cancer or other abnormalities.

These tests are covered services for all women with Medicare. You may receive these services once every 24 months, or every 12 months if:

- You are at high risk for cervical or vaginal cancer (based on your medical history or other findings), or
- You are of childbearing age and have had an abnormal Pap test in the past 36 months

Are you at high risk for cervical cancer? Your risk for cervical cancer increases if:

- You have had an abnormal Pap test
- You have been infected with the human papillomavirus (HPV)
- You began having sex before age 16
- You have had many sexual partners
- You have not had three negative (or any) Pap smears in the past 7 years

Are you at high risk for vaginal cancer? Your risk for vaginal cancer increases if your mother took DES (diethylstilbestrol), a hormonal drug, when she was pregnant with you. In Original Medicare, there is no cost to you for the Pap lab test. For Pap test collection and pelvic and clinical breast exams, you pay 20% of the Medicare-approved amount and no Part B deductible.

PROSTATE CANCER SCREENING

In men, the older you are, the greater your risk of getting and being diagnosed with prostate cancer. The following statistics show the likelihood of being diagnosed with prostate cancer:

- Age 45 – 1 in 2500
- Age 50 – 1 in 476
- Age 55 – 1 in 120
- Age 60 – 1 in 43
- Age 65 – 1 in 21
- Age 70 – 1 in 13
- Age 75 – 1 in 9

Although all men are at risk for prostate cancer, your risk increases if you have a father, brother, or son who has had prostate cancer.

Frequency of Coverage for Prostate Cancer Screenings

Medicare covers screenings for prostate cancer every 12 months for men aged 50 and older. Coverage begins the day after your 50th birthday. The tests in this screening include the prostate-specific antigen (PSA) blood test and a digital rectal examination. You pay 20% of the Medicare-approved amount for the digital rectal examination after the yearly Part B deductible in the Original Medicare Plan. There is no cost for the PSA blood (lab) test.

BREAST CANCER

Breast cancer is the most common nonskin cancer in women and the second leading cause of cancer death in women in the United States.

Every woman is at risk, and this risk increases with age. Breast cancer can usually be successfully treated when found early. Medicare covers screening mammograms to check for breast cancer before you or a doctor may be able to feel it. A mammogram is an x-ray examination of the breast to find any tissue that might not be normal. It is used to look for breast cancer. Medicare coverage includes new digital technology for mammogram screening. A **screening mammogram** is a mammogram of a woman with no signs or symptoms of breast disease. Finding small breast cancers early by a screening mammogram greatly improves a woman's chance for successful treatment. This service is covered for all women with Medicare. You may get one screening mammogram from age 35 to 39 and then one every year starting at age 40. The first mammogram can be used as a baseline to compare with later x-rays. In the Original Medicare Plan, you pay 20% of the Medicare-approved amount, but you do not have to meet the Part B deductible first. You do not need a doctor's referral, but the x-ray supplier will need to send your test results to a doctor.

Up to this point, I have only talked about **screening** mammograms, a preventive Medicare benefit. You should know that Medicare also covers **diagnostic** mammograms. A diagnostic mammogram is used when there are clinical findings, such as a lump that can be felt or an abnormal screening mammogram, that call for additional study. Medicare covers as many diagnostic mammograms as needed. Medicare also covers diagnostic mammograms for men.

Diagnostic mammograms may include additional views of the breast. Medicare pays differently for diagnostic mammograms. Medicare also pays for other diagnostic tests that may be needed, such as an ultrasound.

SMOKING CESSATION

Medicare covers services to help people quit smoking and other tobacco use. The U.S. Surgeon General has reported that quitting smoking leads to significant health benefits, even in older adults who have smoked for years. The benefit covers people with Medicare who have an illness caused or complicated by smoking. This includes smokers with heart or lung disease, stroke, multiple cancers, weak bones, blood clots, or cataracts. Coverage also applies to people taking medications affected by smoking, such as insulin and medicines for high blood pressure, blood clots, and depression. Services can be provided in the hospital or on an outpatient basis. (However, the benefit does not cover hospitalization if tobacco cessation is the primary reason for the hospital stay.)

Medicare will cover two cessation attempts per year. Each attempt may include up to four counseling sessions, with the total annual benefit covering up to eight sessions in a 12-month period. You must get counseling from a qualified Medicare provider (physician, physician assistant, nurse practitioner, clinical nurse specialist, or clinical psychologist). Medicare pays 80% of the cost for these services. Many drugs are available to help you quit smoking, like nicotine patches, and Medicare now covers prescription drugs.

VACCINATIONS

Medicare covers three types of vaccinations. Influenza, also known as the flu, is a contagious disease that is caused by the influenza virus. It attacks the nose, throat, and lungs. The flu is a serious illness that can lead to pneumonia. It can be dangerous for people age 50 and older. You need a flu shot each year because flu viruses are always changing. The shot is updated each year for the most current flu viruses. According to the Centers for Disease Control and Prevention, the flu shot only helps protect you from the flu for about a year. All people with Medicare are eligible for this benefit. You can get a flu shot once each flu season, in the fall or winter. The best time to get a flu shot is in October or November. Avoid getting a flu shot too early because protection from flu can begin to decline within a few months. Flu activity in the United States generally peaks between late December and early March. You can still benefit from getting a flu shot after November, even if the flu is present in your community. You should be able to get the shot any time during the flu season. Once you get a flu shot, your body makes protective antibodies in about 2 weeks. In

Original Medicare, you generally pay nothing for a flu shot, as long as the doctor or nurse accepts Medicare assignment. If you are enrolled in a Medicare Advantage Plan, you generally must see your primary care doctor to get your flu shot, and there may be a copayment for the office visit.

Medicare also covers a vaccination to protect you from pneumococcal pneumonia. Pneumococcal pneumonia is an inflammation in the lungs caused by infection with bacteria called *Streptococcus pneumoniae*. Pneumococcal pneumonia can infect the upper respiratory tract and can spread to the blood, lungs, middle ear, or nervous system. One shot could be all you ever need to protect you from this. All people with Medicare are eligible for this benefit. You pay no coinsurance and no Part B deductible in the Original Medicare Plan if your healthcare provider accepts assignment.

Hepatitis B is a serious disease caused by a virus that inflames the liver. The virus, which is called hepatitis B virus (HBV), can cause lifelong infection, cirrhosis (scarring) of the liver, liver cancer, liver failure, and death. Hepatitis B shots are covered if you are at medium or high risk. Three shots are needed for complete protection. High-risk individuals include those with end-stage renal disease, hemophilia, or a condition that lowers your resistance to infection. (End-stage renal disease is permanent kidney failure that is treated with regular dialysis or a kidney transplant. Hemophilia is a bleeding disorder.) In Original Medicare, you pay 20% of the Medicare-approved amount after the Part B deductible.

Sources of Information on Medicare Preventive Services

There are numerous sources of information on preventive services. The Centers for Medicare and Medicaid Services publishes a brochure called *Medicare Preventive Services to Help Keep You Healthy* (Publication 10110). This brochure is available in English, Spanish, and Chinese, as well as in TTY format. Information on preventive services is also covered in the *Medicare & You* handbook and in *Your Medicare Benefits* (Publication 10116). This publication is available in both English and Spanish. The Medicare helpline is always a source for more information at 1-800-MEDICARE (1-800-633-4227). TTY users should call 1-877-466-2048. Medicare's website (www.medicare.gov) lists other useful sources of preventive service information.

Many of the preventive services are screenings for early detection of cancer. You can get additional information from the American Cancer Society website (www.cancer.org). The toll-free number is 1-800-ACS-2345 (1-800-227-2345). Other information sources include the Centers for Disease Control and Prevention (www.cdc.gov); the Surgeon General's website on tobacco cessation; the National Center for Infectious Diseases (www.cdc.gov/ncidod); and the National Cancer Institutes Cancer Information Service at 1-800-4CANCER (1-800-422-6237), TTY: 1-800-332-8615.

Summary

This chapter has focused on steps you can take to live a longer and healthier life. These steps include taking advantage of the many preventive services covered by Medicare. These services are available whether you are covered by the Original Medicare Plan or a Medicare Advantage or other Medicare plan.

CHAPTER FIFTEEN

Issues That Currently Affect Everyday Medicine Taking

Introduction

This chapter will address issues that currently are receiving a great deal of attention. These issues may affect you now and more than likely will continue to be important issues for a long period of time. Even if you are currently unaffected, chances are good that you know someone or have a relative who has been and will continue to be influenced by these issues.

Off-Label Prescribing

When drugs are approved for use in the United States by the Food and Drug Administration (FDA), they have a defined use for which they are approved. Off-label prescribing can be defined as a drug used for an indication, with a dosage form, dose regimen, population, or other use not mentioned in the approved labeling for the drug product. There is a legally binding agreement between the FDA and the manufacturer to promote (market) the drug for only the defined use. FDA does not regulate the practice of medicine (i.e., "off-label" use); see Section 906 of Federal Food, Drug, and Cosmetic Act. Off-label prescribing is legal and intended to give physicians the flexibility to prescribe the drugs that are best suited to their patients' needs.

Pharmaceutical manufacturers cannot proactively discuss uses or distribute written materials (promotional materials, reprints of studies, etc.) that mention off-label use. However, the FDA does not prohibit others from distributing copies of reprints or reports of off-label uses of drugs.

A University of Georgia study has found that three quarters of people prescribed antidepressant drugs receive the medications for a reason not approved by the Food and Drug Administration (Chen et al, 2006). In this study, my colleagues and I found that 75% of antidepressant recipients, 80% of anticonvulsant recipients, and 64% of antipsychotic recipients received at least one of these medications off label. As previously noted, this practice, known as off-label prescribing, is legal and intended to give physicians the flexibility to prescribe the drugs that are best suited to their patients' needs. I will freely acknowledge that there are legitimate uses for off-label prescribing, but in many cases, physicians write off-label prescriptions based on limited or anecdotal evidence.

Most off-label drug mentions (70–75%) have little or no scientific support. Many patients have no idea that this goes on and just assume that the physician is writing a prescription for their indication.

These findings reveal a significant gap in the nation's drug safety system. The FDA approval process is widely regarded as the world's most rigorous, but off-label prescribing regularly exposes consumers to drugs that are untested for their condition. There is a big gap between this very strict approval process and this very liberal utilization practice. I feel that something must be done to fill this gap.

Off-label use of central nervous system drugs can account for anywhere from 25% to 80% of a drug's annual sales. In the case of the epilepsy and nerve damage drug Neurontin (gabapentin), nearly all patients (98%) received the drug off label in 2001. The drug was commonly prescribed for psychiatric conditions such as bipolar disorder as well as for conditions such as migraine headaches and back pain.

When considering the aging population and the increasing likelihood of off-label prescribing with age, the number of people receiving off-label prescriptions will likely increase in the coming years. The high rate of off-label prescribing for antidepressants likely stems from the high degree of overlap in symptoms among various mental illnesses. The high rates of off-label prescribing of powerful antipsychotic and anticonvulsant drugs for the elderly underscores the lack of effective treatments for Alzheimer's disease and other forms of dementia.

Although off-label prescribing is legal, pharmaceutical companies cannot legally promote an off-label use unless studies support its use.

In 2004, the pharmaceutical company Pfizer paid $430 million and pleaded guilty to a lawsuit that charged its representatives of illegally marketing Neurontin for unapproved uses. Last year, the FDA asked the company to review its data to assess whether Neurontin is linked to suicide attempts. There have been some horror stories recently, one being the case of Neurontin.

I feel that a greater emphasis on evidence-based medicine, which relies on data rather than anecdotal evidence, would ensure greater safety in off-label prescribing. Physicians need to tell their patients when and why they prescribe a drug off label. Physicians have the right to prescribe any medication off label, but they also have the responsibility to inform patients that this medication is being used off label. Patients also need to be their own best advocate and to ask questions about the drugs their doctors prescribe.

There are legitimate uses for off-label prescribing, but knowing this information sets up an opportunity for you to talk to your physician or talk to your pharmacist about exactly why you are being prescribed a drug. I encourage people to do that in all cases and with all drugs.

FDA, Warner-Lambert, and Neurontin

Let's delve deeper into the case concerning the FDA, Warner-Lambert (acquired by Pfizer), and Neurontin. The following is excerpted from an article by the U.S. Food and Drug Administration (2004).

Pharmaceutical manufacturer Warner-Lambert has agreed to plead guilty and pay more than $430 million to resolve criminal charges and civil liabilities in connection with its Parke-Davis division's illegal and fraudulent promotion of unapproved uses for the drug Neurontin (gabapentin). The drug was approved by the Food and Drug Administration in December 1993 solely for use with other drugs to control seizures in people with epilepsy.

Under the provisions of the Federal Food, Drug, and Cosmetic Act, a company must specify the intended uses of a product in its new drug appli-

cation to the FDA. Once approved, the drug may not be marketed or promoted for so-called off-label uses—any use not specified in an application and approved by the FDA.

Warner-Lambert's strategic marketing plans, as well as other evidence, show that Neurontin was aggressively marketed to treat a wide array of ailments for which the drug was not approved, according to a recent press statement from the U.S. Department of Justice. The company promoted Neurontin for the treatment of:

- *bipolar mental disorder*
- *various pain disorders*
- *amyotrophic lateral sclerosis (ALS), commonly referred to as Lou Gehrig's disease*
- *attention-deficit disorder*
- *migraine*
- *drug and alcohol withdrawal seizures*
- *restless leg syndrome*

The company also promoted the drug as a first-line monotherapy treatment for epilepsy (i.e., using Neurontin alone, rather than in addition to another drug).

Warner-Lambert promoted Neurontin even when scientific studies had shown it was not effective. For example, the company promoted Neurontin as effective for use as the sole drug for epileptic seizures, even after solo use had been specifically rejected by the FDA. Similarly, the pharmaceutical company falsely promoted Neurontin as effective for treating bipolar disorder, even when a scientific study demonstrated that a placebo worked as well or better than the drug.

"This illegal and fraudulent promotion scheme corrupted the information process relied upon by doctors in their medical decision-making, thereby putting patients at risk," said U.S. Attorney Michael Sullivan. "This scheme deprived federally-funded Medicaid programs across the country of the informed, impartial judgment of medical professionals—judgment on which the program relies to allocate scarce financial resources to provide necessary and appropriate care to the poor. The pharmaceutical industry will not be allowed to profit from such conduct nor subject the *poor, the elderly, and other persons insured by state and federal healthcare programs to experimental drug uses which have not been determined to be safe and effective."*

As a consequence of the unlawful promotion scheme, patients who received the drug for unapproved and unproven uses had no assurance that their doctors were exercising their independent and fully informed medical judgment or whether the doctor was instead influenced by misleading statements or inducements from Warner-Lambert. Potential problems that can arise from off-label use without the benefit of careful FDA oversight include the occurrence of unforeseen problems because the drug was not studied in the type of patient it is being used for off-label, and the appropriate dosage and course of treatment have not been established.

Warner-Lambert used a number of tactics to achieve its marketing goals, including encouraging sales representatives to provide one-on-one sales pitches to physicians about off-label uses of Neurontin without prior inquiry by doctors. The company's agents also made false or misleading statements to healthcare professionals regarding Neurontin's efficacy and whether it had been approved by the FDA for the off-label uses. Warner-Lambert also used "medical liaisons," who represented themselves (often falsely) as scientific experts in a particular disease, to promote off-label uses for Neurontin.

Warner-Lambert paid doctors to attend so-called "consultants' meetings" in which physicians received a fee for attending expensive dinners or conferences during which presentations about off-label uses of Neurontin were made. These events included lavish weekends and trips to Florida, the 1996 Atlanta Olympics, and Hawaii. There was little or no significant consulting provided by the physicians.

The pharmaceutical company implemented numerous teleconferences in which physicians were recruited by sales representatives to call into a pre-arranged number where they would listen to a doctor or Warner-Lambert employee speak about off-label use of Neurontin. The company also sponsored purportedly "independent medical education" events on off-label Neurontin uses with extensive input from Warner-Lambert regarding topics, speakers, content, and participants.

Warner-Lambert misled the medical community beforehand about the content, as well as the lack of independence from the company's influence, of many of these educational events. In at least one instance, when unfavorable remarks were proposed by a speaker, Warner-Lambert offset the negative impact by "planting" people in the audience to ask questions highlighting the benefits of the drug.

Warner-Lambert paid physicians to allow a sales representative to accompany the physician while he or she saw patients, with the representative offering advice regarding the patient's treatment that was biased toward the use of Neurontin.

These tactics were part of a widespread, coordinated national effort to implement an off-label marketing plan. At the same time, Warner-Lambert decided not to seek FDA approval for any of the new uses because it was concerned that approval for any of the non-epilepsy uses would allow generic competitors of Neurontin to compete with a "son of Neurontin" drug that Warner-Lambert hoped to have approved by the FDA for both epilepsy and non-epilepsy uses.

Neurontin was put on the market in February of 1994. From mid-1995 to at least 2001, the growth of off-label sales was tremendous. While not all of these sales were the consequence of Warner-Lambert's illegal marketing, the marketing scheme was very successful in increasing Neurontin prescriptions for unapproved uses.

The investigation began in the District of Massachusetts when a former medical liaison for Warner-Lambert, David Franklin, M.D., filed suit on behalf of the U.S. government. Private individuals are allowed to file whistleblower suits under the federal False Claims Act to bring the United States information about wrongdoing. If the United States is successful in resolving or litigating the whistleblower's claims, the whistleblower may share part of the recovery. As a part of the resolution, Franklin will receive about $24.6 million of the civil recovery.

The Federal Bureau of Investigation, the Department of Veterans Affairs' Office of Criminal Investigations, the FDA's Office of Criminal Investigations, and the Office of Inspector General for the Department of Health and Human Services conducted the investigation.

Terms of the agreement include:

- *Warner-Lambert has agreed to plead guilty to two counts of violating the Federal Food, Drug, and Cosmetic Act with regard to its misbranding* *of Neurontin by failing to provide adequate directions for use and by introduction into interstate commerce of an unapproved new drug. Warner-Lambert has, as punishment for these offenses, agreed to pay a $240 million criminal fine, the second-largest criminal fine ever imposed in a healthcare fraud prosecution.*

- *Warner-Lambert has agreed to settle its federal civil False Claims Act liabilities and to pay the United States $83.6 million, plus interest, in civil damages for losses suffered by the federal portion of the Medicaid program as a result of Warner-Lambert's fraudulent drug promotion and marketing misconduct.*

- *Warner-Lambert has agreed to settle its civil liabilities to the 50 states and the District of Columbia in an amount of $38 million, plus interest, for harm caused to consumers and to fund a remediation program to address the effects of Warner-Lambert's improper marketing scheme.*

- *Pfizer Inc., Warner-Lambert's parent company, has agreed to comply with the terms of a corporate compliance program, which will ensure that the changes Pfizer Inc. made after acquiring Warner-Lambert in June 2000 are effective in training and supervising its marketing and sales staff.*

FDA Health Advisory for Gabitril

In February of 2005, the FDA released the following Public Health Advisory concerning Gabitril (U.S. Food and Drug Administration, 2005).

Today, the Food and Drug Administration announced that a Bolded Warning will be added to the labeling for Gabitril (tiagabine) to warn prescribers of the risk of seizures in patients without epilepsy being treated with this drug. Gabitril has been approved since 1997 for patients 12 years of age and older as adjunctive therapy (used in addition to other medications) for partial seizures. Recently, the Agency has become aware of reports of the occurrence of seizures in more than 30 patients prescribed Gabitril for conditions other than epilepsy. Most of these uses were in patients with psychiatric illnesses. Such so-called off label *prescribing is a common practice among physicians. Because of the risk of seizures, how–*

ever, in addition to adding the Bolded Warning to product labeling, the sponsor has agreed to undertake an educational campaign targeted to healthcare professionals and patients in which such off label use will be discouraged.

In addition to the occurrence of isolated seizures, the Agency has received several reports of status epilepticus in patients without epilepsy. Status epilepticus is a particularly dangerous event, in which patients have continuous seizures without regaining consciousness between seizures. In some cases, prescribers have continued to treat with, or actually increased the dose of, Gabitril in patients without epilepsy in whom seizures occurred. Presumably, this was done because the prescribers were unaware of the possibility that Gabitril could cause seizures and they believed that, as a drug approved to treat epilepsy, Gabitril might be beneficial in this situation as well.

Typically, the seizures have occurred soon after the initiation of treatment with Gabitril, or soon after an increase in dose, although some patients experienced seizures after several months of treatment. Some seizures have occurred at very low doses compared to the doses approved for use in patients with epilepsy. Although most of the patients in whom seizures occurred were also taking other medications that may infrequently cause seizures, the temporal relationship to the initiation of treatment with Gabitril or to dose increases in many cases, as well as the number of patients reporting seizures, strongly suggests that the seizures were caused by Gabitril.

Because the system for reporting adverse events is voluntary, the number of reports of adverse reactions that the Agency receives once a drug has been marketed is probably less than the actual number of reactions that have actually occurred. For this reason, it is expected that the number of patients who have experienced a seizure while taking Gabitril is likely to be greater than the number reported, although it is impossible to know what the difference might be.

Because seizures are a serious and potentially life-threatening event and because prescribers are unlikely to expect that a drug to treat epilepsy can cause seizures in other patients, the Agency has requested that this information be included in a Bolded Warning and announced to health-care professionals with a Dear Health Care Practitioner letter from the *sponsor. In addition, as noted above, the sponsor has agreed to undertake an educational campaign in which they will discourage the off label use of Gabitril. The Agency will work closely with the sponsor to expedite the adoption and dissemination of the revised label and educational materials.*

Healthcare professionals should be aware that the use of Gabitril for any indication other than for partial seizures in patients with epilepsy who are at least 12 years old is an off label use, meaning evidence to support the safety and effectiveness for those uses has not been approved by the FDA. For this reason, the labeling for Gabitril will not contain any needed precautions and warnings that might result from such a submission and review. Patients should be aware that the use of Gabitril for the treatment of any condition other than partial seizures is considered off label use, and that there is a risk that they may experience a seizure. The risks of seizures should be explained, and patients should report any adverse events promptly to their healthcare professional.

Off-Label Prescribing of Drugs for Cancer

In a 2004 federal agency report (U.S. Department of Health and Human Services, Food and Drug Administration, Center for Drug Evaluation and Research, and Center for Biologics Evaluation and Research, 2004), it was noted that off-label therapy with cancer drugs is common. When there is no established therapy for a cancer or stage of cancer, it is common for oncologists to try different regimens or combinations of established drugs. Cancer drugs are important to consider here because of all the things that oncologists try to implement to help cancer patients as much as possible. Treating oncology patients is an art, and it would simply be impossible for all drug combinations to be tested before they need to be used to help patients.

Special Case of Pediatric Patients

There is inadequate information for approximately three quarters of all pediatric drug use.

Imported Drugs

The high cost of drugs in the United States has forced the attention of many sectors of our country on drugs and their costs. Drugs are being purchased throughout the world and brought into the United States. In Congressional testimony, Dr. Marvin Shepherd from the University of Texas College of Pharmacy noted the problem of counterfeiting and suggested that 25-40% of visitors to Mexico bring back a prescription drug (Shepherd, 2002).

Consumers are faced with an uncertain dilemma regarding the safety of imported drugs and the discrepancy between products obtained from varying countries; this dilemma is compounded by the rapidly increasing price of prescription medications in the United States. Many are forced to make decisions with unfounded beliefs in safety or assumptions regarding the quality of drugs being similar from country to country. An overriding component in all of this is the desire to obtain necessary drugs at reasonable prices.

There have been insistent voices calling for the increased purchase of drugs from Canada as a right. Others are just as adamant that drug importation is not the answer to the high cost of drugs in the United States. Some will point to the risks associated with unknowing importation of counterfeit drugs. The exportation of drugs from Canada to the United States is increasing dramatically from year to year. For example, between 2002 and 2003, the percentage of drugs exported from Manitoba to the United States increased from 24.9% to 40.8% of all sales of all therapeutic class drugs.

The Canadian drug distribution system is meant to supply the needs of 30+ million Canadians and cannot supply drugs to both Canadians and millions in the United States as well. There are 10 times as many prescriptions filled in the United States as there are in Canada.

Another issue regarding the use of drugs from Canada is that American consumers waive their rights of protection under U.S. law before they fill a prescription in a Canadian pharmacy. Before a prescription can be filled in Canada, it must be signed by a Canadian doctor. This places Canadian doctors at risk as well because their malpractice insurance will provide no liability coverage for prescriptions for American patients.

Canada has a strict regulatory control process over drugs (Health Canada) similar to the U.S. Food and Drug Administration (FDA). Other countries may or may not have regulatory control that could be considered equivalent to these systems in the United States and Canada. For example, Mexico does not have a regulatory agency such as the FDA in the United States or Health Canada in Canada.

Health Canada only regulates drugs used in Canada for Canadians. So imported bulk drug supplies that are imported into Canada and exported to the United States are exempt. This is because these imported and exported drugs are not meant for use by Canadian patients. Regulatory authorities responsible for drug oversight in both the United States (FDA) and Canada (Health Canada) have consistently raised safety concerns over personal importation of drugs.

Counterfeit Drugs

Counterfeit drugs are products that do not contain what they are supposed to contain. It is estimated that 10% of the drugs used worldwide are fakes. Unscrupulous criminals are making counterfeiting lucrative for themselves and disastrous for patients. Counterfeiting of prescription drugs was unheard of just a few years ago; unfortunately, however, it is now a commonly discussed issue. Recent Federal Bureau of Investigation (FBI) arrests have highlighted the current issues with counterfeiting of prescription drugs (More arrested in pharmaceutical black market ring, 2004). FBI agents made more arrests in September, 2004 in an operation to dismantle a ring believed responsible for trafficking over $56 million in stolen and counterfeit pharmaceuticals over the past 15 months. Pharmacists were implicated in this operation, so you have to find a pharmacist you can trust and monitor to assure the trust is well placed.

The counterfeiting concern is pressing and unprecedented. It has reached the point where the integrity of the nation's drug supply is suspect. With estimates of counterfeiting occurring 10% of the time, one can understand why. Continuing problems in the future may require drug validation and control by pharmacists in addition to what is in place now. These validations may include the use of color-changing inks and invisible bar coding. Coupled with this important issue of counterfeiting is the unsavory consideration of unscrupulous and unethical pharmacists.

Numerous reasons exist for why counterfeiting has increased in the United States. The upsurge in the number of secondary wholesalers has made it easier for counterfeited drugs to enter the channel of distribution for pharmaceuticals. Secondary wholesalers are ostensibly set up to provide legitimate drugs for sale at reduced prices. In fact, they make an easy entry point for substandard drugs. Increasingly, the type of drugs counterfeited has moved from obscure, expensive drugs to more commonly used drugs at lower price echelons (e.g., Lipitor). Fakes are becoming more sophisticated (e.g., Serostim) in package design and presentation. In addition, unfortunately, the possibility of organized crime and/or terrorist groups playing a role has been suggested. The willful sale of substandard products with adulterated content and the intent to harm can now more easily occur in the United States with imported drugs. The future will see substandard drugs flooding the U.S. market from India and China.

How to Protect Yourself?

Make every effort to know your pharmacist so that you can feel comfortable placing your trust in the individuals who process your prescription orders. Ask your friends and family to recommend a pharmacy that they trust. No doubt, we will see more attention placed, from all levels of our government, on how to ensure that our drugs are what they are supposed to be.

References

Chen H, Kennedy K, Fincham J, Dorfman J, Reeves J, Martin B. Prevalence and factors associated with the off-label use of antidepressant, anticonvulsant and antipsychotic medications among Georgia Medicaid eligibles in 2001. *J Clin Psychiatry* 2006;67:972–982.

More arrested in pharmaceutical black market ring. September 9, 2004. Accessed April 17, 2005. Available at http://www.newsday.com/news/local/wire/ny-bc-nj—thwartingcounterf0909sep09,0,7831306.story?coll=ny-ap-regional-wire.

Shepherd M. Prepared witness testimony. Examining prescription drug importation: A review of a proposal to allow third parties to reimport prescription drugs. Committee on Energy and Commerce, Subcommittee on Health, Washington, DC, U.S. Government Printing Office: 112, 2002.

U.S. Department of Health and Human Services, Food and Drug Administration, Center for Drug Evaluation and Research, and Center for Biologics Evaluation and Research. Guidance for industry IND exemptions for studies of lawfully marketed drug or biological products for the treatment of cancer. 2004. Available at http://www.fda.gov/cder/guidance/6036fnl.htm; accessed March 22, 2007.

U.S. Food and Drug Administration. Drug maker to pay $430 million in fines, civil damages. 2004. Available at http://www.fda.gov/fdac/features/2004/404_wl.html; accessed March 22, 2007.

U.S. Food and Drug Administration. FDA Public Health Advisory: Seizures in patients without epilepsy being treated with Gabitril (tiagabine). February 18, 2005. Available at http://www.fda.gov/cder/drug/advisory/gabitril.htm; accessed March 22, 2007.

Websites for Senior Citizen Information

Specific Websites with Information of Use to Seniors, Families, and Caregivers about Medicare Part D

Centers for Medicare and Medicaid Services:
- Information about prescription drug plans and coverage issues: http://www.cms.hhs.gov/PrescriptionDrugCovGenIn/03_Resource.asp#TopOfPage
- General information about prescription drug coverage: http://www.cms.hhs.gov/PrescriptionDrugCovGenIn/
- Comparing various plans, examining your current plan: http://www.medicare.gov/MPDPF

Medicare Education: www.medicareeducation.org

Social Security Administration website: www.ssa.gov

The National Council on Aging—NCOA is a national voice and powerful advocate for public policies that promote vital aging. website: http://www.ncoa.org

Access to Benefits Coalition—Rx access for those who need them most. There are currently more than 70 national non-profit members of the Access to Benefits Coalition, who share the interest of helping low-income Medicare beneficiaries find the public and private prescription savings programs they need to maintain their health and improve the quality of their lives. website: http://www.accesstobenefits.org

Various Helpful Resources on Prescription Programs That Help Seniors Save Money

www.crbestbuydrugs.org/: Contains important information from Consumer Reports about saving money on prescription drugs.

www.ashp.org/pap/: Created by the American Society of Health-System Pharmacists with support from the Health Resources and Services Administration. Provides information on patient assistance programs.

www.eldercare.gov: Run by the U.S. Administration on Aging. Shows drug assistance programs by state. Phone: (800) 677-1116.

www.gskforyou.com/index.htm: GlaxoSmithKline Pharmaceutical Company patient assistance website.

www.needymeds.com: Lists information about state programs, discount drug cards, federal poverty guidelines, and patient assistance programs and includes copies of the forms.

www.rxassist.com: Run by Volunteers in Health Care. Allows searches by medicine and manufacturer, and helps find assistance programs nationwide.

www.helpingpatients.org: A resource for patient assistance programs. Run by the Pharmaceutical Research and Manufacturers of America.

www.merckhelps.com: A resource for patient assistance programs. Provided by Merck and Company.

General Health Information Sources

WebMD Health
- http://my.webmd.com/medical_information/condition_centers/default.htm
- http://my.webmd.com/medical_information/medicare_rx_benefits/default.htm

The Mayo Clinic: http://www.mayoclinic.com/index.cfm

United States Government Healthfinder–affiliated organizations and websites: http://www.healthfinder.gov/organizations/

Several Disease–Based National Organization Websites

American Heart Association: http://www.americanheart.org

American Diabetes Association: http://www.diabetes.org

American Cancer Society: http://www.cancer.org

American Lung Association: http://www.lungusa.org

Websites Especially Designed for Women

http://www.womens-health.org/consumers.htm

http://www.4woman.gov/

Websites for More Information about Drugs

Before I list the specific websites I would like to provide here, I want to say a little about websites and information that appears on the internet. Not everything that is on a website is accurate information. Some of what appears is not worth reading and certainly is suspect in the accuracy of the materials presented. There is a foundation called Health on the Net (HON) that will help guide you to accurate information. The mission of HON, as stated on their website:

"is to guide the growing community of healthcare consumers and providers on the World Wide Web to sound, reliable medical information and expertise. In this way, HON seeks to contribute to better, more accessible and cost-effective health care."

If the website that you are examining has the seal of approval from HON, then it lets you know that the site has been evaluated for accuracy. HON provides a code of conduct for Web information. It can be found at: http://www.hon.ch/HONcode/Conduct.html.

I will recommend only those sites that provide unbiased drug information for consumers. Many websites provide drug information but do so to encourage the consumer to purchase medications online.

National Library of Medicine and National Institutes of Health (both Spanish and English versions):
- http://www.nlm.nih.gov/medlineplus/druginformation.html
- http://medlineplus.gov/esp/

The Mayo Clinic: http://www.mayoclinic.com/index.cfm

The Herbal Research Foundation supports a website with comprehensive information about herbs and herbal supplements: http://www.herbs.org/

The United States Food and Drug Administration website for consumer education and information: http://www.fda.gov/cder/consumerinfo/DPAdefault.htm

- The FDA is committed to providing consumers with information on prescription, generic, and over-the-counter drug products. The Center for Drug Evaluation and Research has developed numerous public service campaigns and announcements to help you make informed decisions about using medicines.

U.S. FDA website on the dangers of mixing drugs and alcohol: http://www.asyouage.samhsa.gov/Default.aspx

U.S. FDA website on several drugs that should not be purchased from non-U.S. sources: http://www.fda.gov/cder/consumerinfo/ dontBuyonNet.htm

Consumer Information from Other Government Agencies

Agency for Healthcare Research and Quality:
- http://www.ahcpr.gov/consumer/5steps.htm
- http://www.healthfinder.gov/

U.S. FDA website for information on nutritional supplements: http://vm.cfsan.fda.gov/~dms/supplmnt.html

U.S. FDA resource for buying drugs online: www.fda.gov/ buyonline

U.S. FDA resource on medication safety: www.fda.gov/cder/ consumerinfo/DPAdefault.htm

Index

www.ingramcontent.com/pod-product-compliance
Lightning Source LLC
Chambersburg PA
CBHW072123020426
42334CB00018B/1696